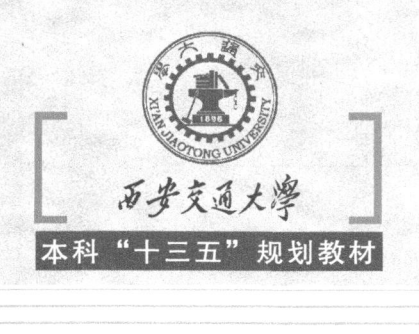

西安交通大学
本科"十三五"规划教材

The Operating Instructions of Regional Anatomy

主　编　董炜疆

副主编　钱亦华　李月英

编　者　杨蓬勃　靳　辉　冯改丰
　　　　肖新莉　董炜疆　钱亦华
　　　　李月英　贾　宁

U0282101

西安交通大学出版社
XI'AN JIAOTONG UNIVERSITY PRESS

图书在版编目(CIP)数据

局部解剖操作指导＝The Operating Instructions
of Regional Anatomy：英文/董炜疆主编. —西安：
西安交通大学出版社,2018.5
西安交通大学本科"十三五"规划教材
ISBN 978－7－5693－0642－2

Ⅰ.①局…　Ⅱ.①董…　Ⅲ.①局部解剖学-高等学校
-教材-英文　Ⅳ.①R323

中国版本图书馆 CIP 数据核字(2018)第 109316 号

书　　名	The Operating Instructions of Regional Anatomy
主　　编	董炜疆
责任编辑	宋伟丽　杜玄静
出版发行	西安交通大学出版社
	(西安市兴庆南路 10 号　邮政编码 710049)
网　　址	http://www.xjtupress.com
电　　话	(029)82668357　82667874(发行中心)
	(029)82668315(总编办)
传　　真	(029)82668280
印　　刷	西安日报社印务中心
开　　本	787mm×1092mm　1/16　印张 12　字数 276 千字
版次印次	2018 年 11 月第 1 版　2018 年 11 月第 1 次印刷
书　　号	ISBN 978－7－5693－0642－2
定　　价	46.00 元

Preface

Human Anatomy is an important basic course for medical students. It is composed of several different subdivisions, among them, regional anatomy is the most important part. It is the study of regions and divisions of the body, and mainly focuses on the relations between various structures, such as muscles, nerves, arteries and so on.

This book is designed to meet the requirements not only for the native students who are using English, but also for those foreign students coming to China for medical education. It is compiled as a supplementary book of The Text Book of Regional Anatomy, so they are the same in the order of chapters. In the laboratory, you will have the chance to know the real body which is full of surprise, and you will get it especially when you dissect the body by yourself based on the instructions.

The operating instructions contain the following parts, reviewing, dissecting and observing, clinical application and asking yourself. They are all organized carefully in order to help students familiar with body dissection, it also encourages the students to explore more medical knowledge during the spare time. And we are sure this book is much like a lighthouse, it tells students where they are and guides them where to go.

During many years of teaching, the authors have never experienced to work with such an effective and well-informed editing group, we spent a year compiling, checking and correcting the book over and over again. We received strong comments and suggestions from our respected colleagues. The authors would also like to thank all professors, teachers and technologists from the Department of Human Anatomy in the Basic Medical Sciences in Xi'an Jiaotong University.

This book is also suitable for those graduated students in the major of Clinical Medicine, it can be a handbook or reference for medical researchers.

Oversights and deficiencies may appear in the book, any corrections and suggestions are greatly appreciated.

C ONTENTS

The Operating Instructions of Regional Anatomy

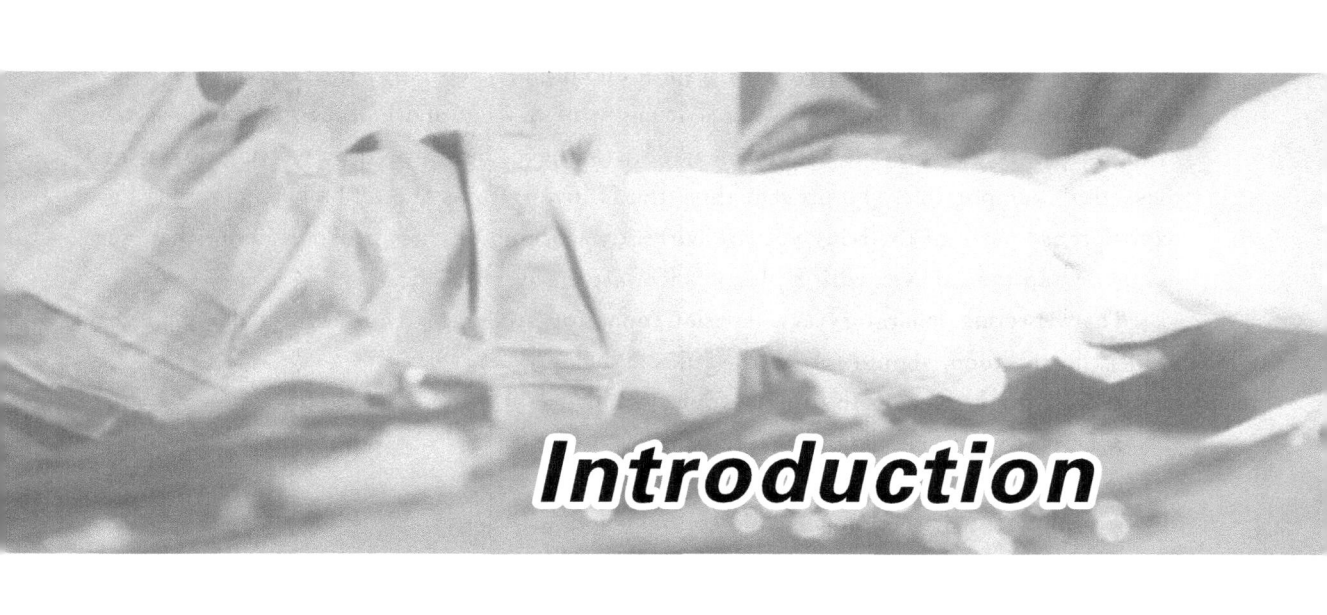

Introduction

The human body consists of the major parts which include head, neck and trunk, and paired upper limbs and lower limbs. Each major part can be further subdivided into several regions. **Regional anatomy** investigates the body's structure located in a particular part or region.

The necessary and most effective way to study the regional anatomy is **cadaver** dissection. Each student should regard the opportunity to dissect the cadaver as a rare privilege. And the cadaver must be treated with respect and dignity. Usually, the cadavers have been kept moist or wet by preservative fluid, it might be dry out and become hard to dissect by evaporation. If a part of the body dries out, it can never be restored by wetting down, and dissection is impossible. To prevent this, the following rules should be kept in mind: only expose those parts of the body you are currently working on, never expose more than necessary; wrap the cadaver with a plastic sheet after each dissection.

The dissecting laboratory is a special room for students to dissect the body. Every student in the room should follow the rules as below:
- Wear long lab coat to protect your clothing.
- Do not wear sandals or open-toe shoes.
- Read the textbook before the dissecting.
- Follow the dissection schedule and instructions.
- Keep the lab clean and tidy.
- All scraps of anatomical material should be put in the provided container.

Dissection instruments

Forceps　There are two kinds of forceps in dissecting. One has tips that are blunt and rounded, and the gripping surfaces are corrugated. It is used to lift and hold vessels, nerves and other structures. It also be used while blunt dissection. The other forceps have teeth. It is used in cutting and grasping the skin (skinning).

Scissors　Scissors are used in cutting and blunt dissection. For blunt dissection, insert the tips of closed scissors into connective tissue and then open, it can tear the connective tissue. This is an effective way to dissect vessels and nerves.

Scalpel　Scalpel is usually used in cutting, removing the superficial fascia and cutting the deep fascia(clean the muscle). It is also used in sharp dissection of cutaneous nerves and superficial blood vessels in the superficial fascia.

Basic structures of human body and basic method for dissection

Skin　The skin is the first layer of human body. Before dissecting, mark out the line of the incision by scratching the skin with the back of the scalpel. Hold the blade at right angle to the skin, drive its point through the skin. Then incline the blade to an angle of 45 to the surface, and carry it steadily to the other end of the lien of incision. Grip the cutting edge(or a convenient angle) of the skin with the forceps, carefully peel back the skin flap.

Superficial fascia   It is a fibrous, fatty covering that underlies the skin, which also called the subcutaneous tissue or subcutaneous fat. The thickness varies due to individuals and regions. It is usually thick in women and childen. The thinnest part in body is the eyelids. After peeling off the skin, observe the thickness of the superficial fascia. Then, look for the cutaneous nerves and superficial vessels, lymph nodes(only in some region) based on their position. There are two ways to dissect this layer: blunt dissection with two forceps or with scissors. Sharp dissection with scalpel. After finding the superficial structures, remove the superficial fascia with the scalpel. Preserve the main cutaneous nerves and main trunk of blood vessels in cadaver carefully.

Deep fascia   Deep fascia is also called the proper fascia that lies beneath the superficial fascia. Observe the deep fascia and identify the structures formed by it. Deep fascia may form sheaths of the muscles and affording them broad surfaces for attachment. In the limbs, it invests the entire limb, and gives off the septa (intermuscular septa) to separate the muscles in groups. It also forms the neurovascular sheaths. At the wrist and ankle, parts of the deep fascia become thick and form the retinaculum to hold the tendons in position.

Muscle   After cutting and removing the deep fascia, skeletal muscles are exposed. The skeletal muscle contains belly and tendons. Clean and separate the muscle, observe its shape and origin, insertion. Try to find blood vessels and nerves which supply the related muscle.

Blood vessels and nerves   Look for and clean the blood vessels and nerves with scissors or scalpel. Identify them according to their shape, position and course. The arteries are thick-walled elastic tubes. The veins are wider and thinner than their accompanying arteries. Nerves are white cords and branched like the arteries. Trace them to their trunk or branches.

Look for and observe the lymph nodes   The lymph nodes are small round or oval shaped bodies alongside the greater blood vessels.

The technique of dissection requires patience and skills. With practice, students will get not only the knowledge, but also the abilities.

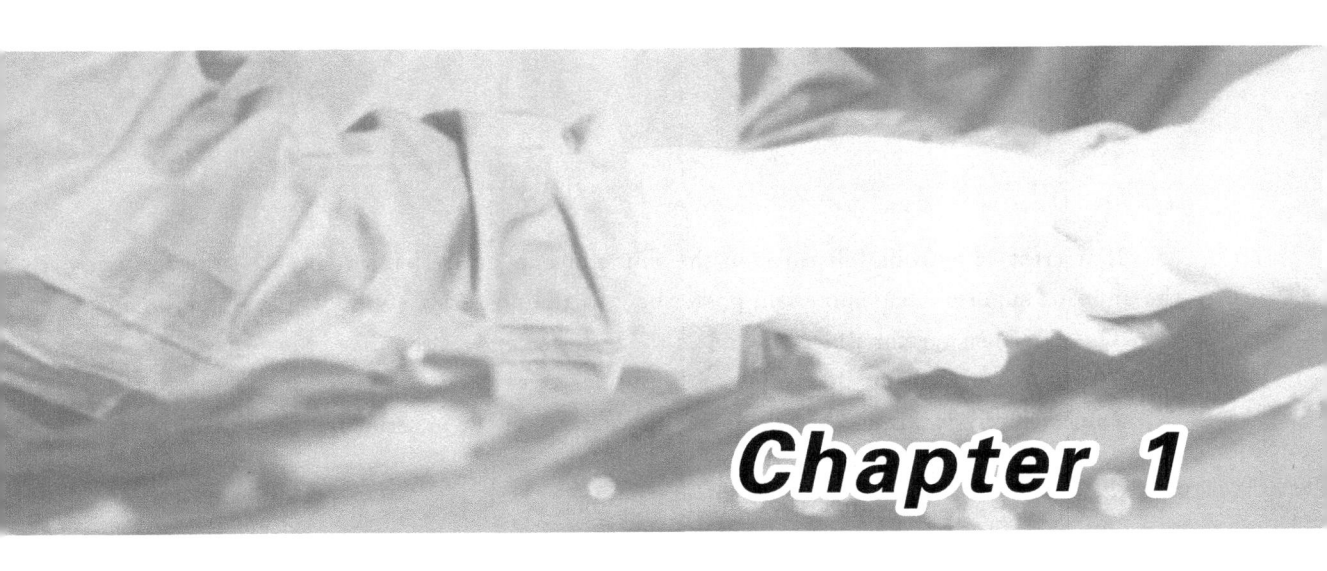

Chapter 1

The lower limb

Section 1   Review

Iliac crest   It can be felt through the skin along its entire length, it ends anteriorly as the anterior superior iliac spine and posteriorly as the posterior superior iliac spine.

The **anterior superior iliac spine**   It's the anterior end of the iliac crest.

The **posterior superior iliac spine**   It's the posterior end of the iliac crest.

Pubic symphysis   It can be felt at the inferior end of the anterior median line of the abdomen.

Pubic crest   It's the upper border of the pubis.

Pubic tubercle   The pubic crest ends laterally as pubic tubercle.

Inguinal ligament   It lies between the anterior surface of the thigh and abdomen.

Ischial tuberosity   It can be easily palpated medially in the lower part of gluteal region as the hip joint flexed, and it forms the posterior aspect of the body of ischium.

Greater trochanter   It can be felt laterally in the middle part of the gluteal region, and it is about 10 cm behind the iliac tubercle.

Patella   It locates in the front of the knee.

Medial and lateral condyles of femur   It lies at the medial and lateral side of patella.

The **tendon of biceps femoris**   It's on the lateral side of the knee and can be felt posteriorly to the head of the fibula when the knee is bent.

The **tendons of semitendinosus and semimembranosus**   It's on the medial side of the knee when the knee is bent.

Patellar ligament   It can be felt below the patella and it is formed by the tendon of the quadriceps femoris.

Head of fibula   It can be felt as a knob of bone and lies the lateral side of the knee.

Shaft of the tibia   It is subcutaneous and readily felt from the tibial tuberosity to the anterior margin of the medial malleolus.

Medial and lateral malleolus   They are the projections of the lower end of the tibia and the fibula respectively.

Calcaneal tuberosity   It is on the posterior of ankle joint and below the tendon calcaneus.

Ⅱ. Boundaries and divisions

It is bounded anteriorly by the inguinal groove that connected with abdomen, and posteriorly by the iliac crest that connected with the waist and sacrum. Between the medial side of the upper extremities of the two limbs is the perineum.

Ⅲ. Main contents

1　Skin

The anterior part of skin is thin, especially on the dorsum of the foot; while the posterior part of skin is thicker, especially on the soles, and skin keratosis of the soles is obvious.

2　Superficial fascia

Also called subcutaneous tissue, it is loose and has the different thickness. It is rich in superficial veins, superficial lymph nodes, lymphatic vessels, cutaneous nerves, etc.

2.1　Superficial veins

● Great saphenous vein　It begins on the medial side of the dorsum of the foot, runs upward anteriorly to the medial malleolus and then on the medial surface of the leg, accompanying with the saphenous nerve. It ascends on the posteromedial surface of the knee and inclines anteriorly through the thigh to enter the femoral vein through the saphenous hiatus. On its course, the great saphenous vein receives superficial veins of the leg and other five tributaries—the superficial lateral femoral vein, the superficial medial femoral vein, the superficial iliac circumflex vein, the superficial epigastric vein and the external pudendal vein.

● Small saphenous vein　It arises from the dorsal venous arch of the foot and ascends behind the lateral malleolus in company with the sural nerve. It runs upward along the midline of the back of the leg to the lower part of the popliteal fossa, where it pierces the deep fascia and ends in the popliteal vein.

2.2　Superficial inguinal lymph nodes

● Upper nodes　They are distal to the inguinal ligament, and they receive the lymph from the skin and superficial tissue of abdominal wall below the level of the umbilicus, the gluteal region, the external genital organs, the perineum and the lower part of the anal canal.

● Lower nodes　They are placed along both sides of the upper part of the great saphenous vein, and they receives the lymph from the superficial structure of the lower limb excluding the lateral part of the foot and heel.

2.3 Cutaneous nerves

2.3.1 Anterior and medial region of the thigh

The lateral femoral cutaneous nerve originats from the lumbar plexus and distributes on the skin of the lateral and anterior surface of the thigh. Anterior cutaneous branches of the femoral nerve are known as the medial and intermediate femoral cutaneous nerves which pierce the deep fascia along an oblique line that corresponding to the direction of the sartorius muscle and supply the skin of the anterior and medial surface of the thigh and of the anterior surface of the knee joint. The cutaneous branches of obturator nerve distributes in the middle and upper surface of the medial thigh.

2.3.2 Anterior lateral region of the leg and dorsum of the foot

The saphenous nerve, which is the terminal branch of the femoral nerve, passes down along the medial side of the leg and accompanies the great saphenous vein to the dorsum of the foot. It supplies the skin on the anteromedial surface of the leg and medial side of the foot. The superficial peroneal nerve becomes cutaneous by piercing the deep fascia in the lateral distal third of the leg and supplies the skin of the lower part of the anterolateral surface of the leg. The lateral dorsal cutaneous nerve of foot, which is the terminal branch of the sural nerve, supplies the skin along the lateral margin of the foot and the lateral side of the little toe.

2.3.3 Gluteal region

The superior gluteal cutaneous nerves are two or three branches of dorsal ramus of upper three lumbar nerve and supply the upper half of the buttock. The inferior gluteal cutaneous nerves which are the gluteal branches of the posterior femoral cutaneous nerve, curve around the lower border of the gluteus maximus to supply the lower part of the buttock. The medial gluteal cutaneous nerves supply the medial part of the buttock.

2.3.4 Posterior thigh

The posterior femoral cutaneous nerve, which derives from the sacral plexus, distributes in the posterior region of thigh and popliteal fossa.

2.3.5 Posterior leg

The medial sural cutaneous nerve from the tibial nerve arises in the popliteal fossa, descends between the two heads of gastrocnemius and pierces the deep fascia in the middle or upper back part of the leg. The lateral sural cutaneous nerve is a branch of the common peroneal nerve, it supplies the skin on the upper part of the posterolateral surface of the leg. The sural nerve which formed by the union of the medial sural cutaneous nerve and the communicating branch of the common peroneal nerve, supplies the skin on the lower part of the posterolateral surface of the leg.

3 Deep fascia

The deep fascia which envelops the muscle, blood vessels and nerves, passes through the muscles to attach the periosteum and forms intermuscular septa and vascular nerve sheath. The deep fascia of the anterior part of the thigh is called the fascia lata. A thickened band occurs on the lateral side of the thigh and is known as the iliotibial tract. Around the ankle joint, the deep fascia thickens to form a support band to fix the muscular tendons.

4 Muscles and deep structures

4.1 Anterior medial femoral region

4.1.1 Muscles

The anterior group includes the quadriceps femoris and the sartorius. The medial group consists of pectineus, adductor longus, gracilis, adductor brevis and adductor magnus.

4.1.2 Deep structures

▶ Lacuna musculorum and lacuna vasorum

The gap between the inguinal ligament and hip bone is divided into the lacuna musculorum laterally and lacuna vasorum medially by the iliopectineal arch.

● Lacuna musculorum It is bounded by the inguinal ligament anteriorly, the ilium posterolaterally, the iliopectineal arch medially. It transmits the iliopsoas, the femoral nerve and the lateral femoral cutaneous nerve.

● Lacuna vasorum It is bounded by the inguinal ligament anteriorly, the pectineal ligament posteriorly, the iliopectineal arch laterally, and the lacunar ligament medially. It transmits the femoral vessels, the femoral canal and the lymphatic vessels.

▶ Femoral triangle

It lies at the superomedial part of the thigh.

● Boundaries Superiorly it is bounded by the inguinal ligament, medially by the medial border of the adductor longus, laterally by the medial border of the sartorius. The roof of triangle is formed by the skin, superficial fascia and fascia lata. The floor of the triangle is formed by the adductor longus, pectineus and iliopsoas.

● Contents They are the femoral nerve, femoral artery, femoral vein, femoral sheath and femoral canal, and deep inguinal lymph nodes which located in the femoral canal.

The femoral nerve arises from the lumbar plexus, descends behind the iliac fascia and enters the femoral triangle posteriorly to the inguinal ligament and laterally to the femoral sheath. Its muscular branches supply the pectineus, the sartorius and the quadriceps femoris. Its articular branches supply the hip and knee joints. Its cutaneous branches are the anterior cutaneous branches and the saphenous nerve.

The femoral artery is continuous with the external iliac artery at the mid-inguinal point, then passing downward to the femoral triangle and enters the adductor canal. The main branch of the femoral artery is the deep femoral artery and its branches (the lateral and medial femoral circumflex artery and three or four perforating arteries).

The femoral vein is medial to the femoral artery, and its tributaries accompany with the branches of the femoral artery, but the great saphenous vein has no counterpart.

The femoral sheath It is formed by the prolongation of the fascia lining the abdomen (transverse fascia anteriorly and iliac fascia posteriorly). The sheath is subdivided by two partitions into three compartments which contain the femoral artery, the femoral vein and the femoral canal from lateral to medial side.

The femoral canal is medial compartments of the femoral sheath which is about 1.5 cm long. The femoral canal contains lymphatic nodes, vessels, loose areolar tissue and fat. The superior opening is called femoral ring. The boundaries of the femoral ring are: the femoral vein, laterally; the pectineal ligament, posteriorly; medially, the inguinal ligament, the lacunar ligament and conjoined tendon (inguinal falx) anteriorly. The femoral canal is the predilection site of femoral hernia which is more common in women.

▶ Adductor canal

It is about 1.5 cm long furrow on the medial side of the midthigh. It starts at the apex of the femoral triangle and ends in the adductor tendinous opening of the adductor magnus. It is bounded anteriorly by the sartorius and the adductor lamina, laterally by the vastus medialis and posteriorly by the adductor longus and the adductor magnus. There are the saphenous nerve, the femoral artery and femoral vein from anterior to posterior in the canal.

4.2 Anterior and lateral region of the leg

4.2.1 Muscles

The anterior group includes tibialis anterior, extensor hallucis longus and extensor digitorum longus. The lateral group consists of the peroneus longus and brevis.

4.2.2 Nerves

The deep peroneal nerve and the superficial peroneal nerve are the terminal branches of the common peroneal nerve. The deep peroneal nerve distributes to the muscles of the anterior group of leg and small muscles of the foot dorsum. The superficial peroneal nerve distributes to the muscles of the lateral group of leg. The anterior tibial artery arises from the popliteal artery and passes forward into the anterior compartment between the tibialis anterior and extensor hallucis longus, accompanying by the deep peroneal nerve and two corresponding veins. In front of the ankle joint, it becomes the dorsal artery of the foot. The anterior tibial artery supplies the muscles of the compartment, knee and ankle joint.

4.3 Gluteal region

4.3.1 Muscles

The muscles can be divided into three layers. The superficial layer consists of the tensor fasciae latae and gluteus maximus. The middle layer are the gluteus medius, piriformis, gemellus superior, tendon of obturator internus, gemellus inferior and the quadrates femoris. The deep layer are the gluteus minimus and the obturator externus.

4.3.2 Deep structures

▶ Suprapiriform foramen

From the lateral to the medidl side, it passes through the superior gluteal nerve, the superior gluteal artery and vein.

▶ Infrapiriform foramen

From the lateral to the medial side, it passes through the sciatic nerve, the posterior femoral cutaneous nerve, the inferior gluteal nerve, the inferior gluteal artery and vein, the internal pudendal artery and vein and the pudendal nerve.

The sciatic nerve is a branch of the sacral plexus, leaves the pelvis through the infrapiriform foramen, passes midway between the greater trochanter and the ischial tuberosity, superficially to the quadratus femoris, then runs downward into the back of the thigh. It is the largest nerve in the body and consists of the tibial and common peroneal nerves bounded together with fascia. The two nerves usually detach from each other one third of the thigh, but occasionally they are separated when they leave the pelvis. In such cases, the common peroneal nerve may pierce the piriformis and pass through the suprapiriform foramen or divide into several division. The sciatic nerve usually has no branches in the gluteal region.

▶ Lesser sciatic foramen

It is the passageway between the gluteal region and the perineum for the internal pudendal artery and vein, pudendal nerve.

4.4 Posterior region of the thigh and leg

4.4.1 Muscles

The muscles of the back of thigh are the biceps femoris on the lateral side, the superficial semitendinosus and deep semimembranosus on the medial side. The muscles of the back of the leg are divided into the superficial and deep group. The superficial group includes the gastrocnemius and soleus. The deep group consists of the flexor digitorum longus, tibialis posterior and flexor hallucis longus.

4.4.2 Deep structures

▶ Popliteal fossa

It is a diamond shaped intermuscular space situated at the back of the knee.

● Boundaries   The upper lateral boundary is formed by the biceps femoris and the upper medial boundary by the semitendinosus and semimembranosus. The lower lateral boundary is formed by the lateral head of the gastrocnemius and the lower medial boundary by the medial head of the gastrocnemius. The floor of the fossa is formed by the popliteal surface of femur, the posterior wall of joint capsule of the knee joint and the popliteus with its fascia. The roof of the popliteal fossa is formed by the popliteal fascia.

● Contents   The tibial nerve and common peroneal nerve, popliteal vein, popliteal artery. In addition, there are some popliteal lymph nodes and fatty connective tissues around above contents.

The tibial nerve lies in the center of the fossa. It passes through the soleus tendon arch and descends between the muscles of the superficial deep layer. It gives off the cutaneous branch (medial sural cutaneous nerve), muscle branches (the muscles of the posterior group) and articulatory branch (knee joint).

The common peroneal nerve lies at the lateral margin of the popliteal fossa. It descends to the fibular neck and divides into the superficial peroneal and deep peroneal nerve. Its another branch is the lateral sural cutaneous nerve.

The popliteal vein is located between the popliteal artery and the tibial nerve.

The popliteal artery, as a continuation of the femoral artery, it lies deeply when enters the popliteal fossa through the adductor tendinous opening. It ends at the level of the lower border of the popliteus by dividing into anterior and posterior tibial arteries.

The popliteal lymph nodes lie along the sheath of popliteal vessel, and collect lymph of the lateral side of foot skin, the lateral half back of the leg, the deep lymphatic vessels of leg and foot. The efferent vessels accompanying the femoral blood vessels end in the deep inguinal lymph nodes.

▶ Malleolar canal

It locates in the medial part of the ankle and is formed by the flexor retinaculum and calcaneus. From anterior to posterior is: the tendon and synovial sheath of the tibialis posterior, the tendon and synovial sheath of the flexor digitorum longus, the posterior tibial nerve, and the tendon and synovial sheath of the flexor hallucis longus.

4.5   The sole of the foot

The muscles can be divided into four layers.

The first layer is the abductor hallucis, flexor digitorum brevis and abductor digiti minimi.

The second layer is the tendon and synovial sheath of flexor digitorum longus, quadratus plantae, lumbricales and the tendon and synovial sheath of flexor hallucis longus.

The third layer is the flexor hallucis brevis, adductor hallucis and flexor digiti minimi brevis.

The fourth layer is the tendons of the peroneus, the tibialis posterior and seven interossei.

Section 2

Dissection and observation

1 Position and incisions

The cadaver is placed in the supine position. Make the following incisions:

● Make an oblique incision from the anterior superior iliac spine to the pubic tubercle along the line of the inguinal ligament.

● Along the pubic tubercle downward and posteriorly to the medial surface of the thigh just skirting the external genital organs, and then make a vertical incision along the medial surface of the thigh to a point that is at the level of the tibial tuberosity.

● Make a transverse incision around the upper part of the leg, starting at the lower end of the above incision.

● Make a vertical incision along the anterior margin of the tibial, from the above transverse incision to the midline of the dorsum of foot.

● Make a curved incision at the level of the malleolus.

● Make a transverse incision at the root of toes.

● Make a incision along the midline of the middle toe.

2 Procedures

Turn the anterior skin flap laterally to hinge on the lateral border of the thigh, pay attention to the cutaneous nerves and vessels especially in the inguinal and knee region. Turn over the skin flap medially and laterally of the medial regions of the leg and dorsum of the foot.

2.1 Dissect the superficial fascia

2.1.1 Find and clean the great saphenous vein and its tributaries

Trace the vein downward to the medial side of the knee and upward to the point where it turns sharply backward through the deep fascia to enter the femoral vein. Identify the tributaries of the great saphenous vein near its upper end, namely, the superficial lateral

— 13 —

femoral vein, the superficial medial femoral vein, the superficial iliac circumflex vein, the superficial epigastric vein and the external pudendal vein.

2.1.2   Observe the superficial inguinal lymph nodes

They can be divided into horizontal and vertical groups. The horizontal group is about one finger's breadth below the inguinal ligament, and the vertical group locates in the terminal part of the great saphenous vein.

2.1.3   Dissect the superficial fascia of the leg and dorsum of the foot

Identify the dorsal venous arch on the dorsum of the foot. The great saphenous vein and small saphenous vein arise from it. On the medial side of the arch, identify the great saphenous vein and follow it upward anteriorly to the medial malleolus and medial aspects of the leg. On the lateral side, find the small saphenous vein and follow it upward posterior to the lateral malleolus.

2.1.4   Dissect the cutaneous nerves

Try to find: ① the lateral femoral cutaneous nerve which is 5-10 cm below the anterior superior iliac spine; ② the ilioinguinal nerve and the femoral branch of genitofemoral nerve; ③ the intermediate femoral cutaneous nerve; ④ the medial femoral cutaneous nerve;⑤ the saphenous nerve appears behind the saphenous vein at the medial side of the knee.

2.2   Examine the deep fascia and expose the deep structure

Preserve the great saphenous vein and its tributaries, cutaneous nerves and dorsal venous arch of foot, remove the remains of the superficial facia.

Observe the cribriform fascia and saphenous hiatus, pay attention to iliotibial tract which is formed by the thickened fascia lata in the lateral region of the thigh. Observe the extensor retinaculum and its attachment.

Clean the boundary of the femoral triangle and examine the contents of the femoral sheath. ① Clean the sartorius which forms the lateral boundary of the triangle downward to the point where it crosses the adductor longus. Clean the adductor longus downward to the point where it disappears behind the sartorius. The medial border of adductor longus forms the medial boundary of the triangle. The inguinal ligament forms the upper boundary of the triangle. ② Remove the adipose tissue below the inguinal ligament carefully to expose the femoral sheath. With the handle of a scalpel, isolate the sheath from the inguinal ligament, understand that it is a downward protrusion into the thigh of the fascia lining the abdominal walls and that it fuses with the coats of the femoral vessels about the level of the lower margin of the saphenous hiatus. ③ Open the femoral sheath by three vertical incisions through its anterior wall: the first covers the femoral artery, the second covers the femoral vein, and the third is a little medial to the vein. Note that the sheath is divided into three compartments. The lateral one is occupied by the femoral artery. The middle one is occupied by the femoral vein. ④ The medial but important compartment is occupied by connective tissue, constant lymph node and lymphatic vessels. It is called the femoral canal. Put your little finger in the canal and insert gently upward to the upper opening of the canal. This opening is called the femoral ring. Define its boundaries with your finger tip. ⑤ Clean and expose the branches of the femoral artery. ⑥ Clean the femoral vein. ⑦ Identify the femoral nerve and branches. The femoral nerve and its branches (muscular branches and anterior cutaneous branches) can be found on the surface of the psoas muscle, trace downward its terminal branch-the saphenous nerve.

2.2.1 Dissect the adductor canal

On the middle one third of the thigh, pull the sartorius laterally. Open the adductor canal by cutting through a strong aponeurosis, the adductor lamina. This lamina is stretched between the vastus medialis anteriorly and the adductor magnus posteriorly. Examin the femoral artery, the femoral vein, the saphenous nerve and their relation.

2.2.2 Observe the quadriceps femoris

Transect the rectus femoris in the middle and reflect upward and downward respectively to expose the vastus intermedius and the branches of the lateral circumflex femoral artery. Trace the rectus femoris, the vastus medialis, the vastus intermedius to their insertion. Note that the tendon is continuous inferiorly to the tibial tuberosity as the patellar ligament.

2.2.3 Dissect the medial part of the thigh

Clean and observe the pectineus, adductor longus and gracilis muscle. Cut the adductor longus near its origin and turn it downward. Find the adductor brevis, the anterior and posterior branch of the obturator nerve and accompanying vessels. In the lower segment of adductor magnus, observe the adductor tendinous opening which transmit the femoral vessels from the adductor canal to the popliteal fossa.

On the lateral side of the tibial shaft, dissect the tibialis anterior, extensor hallucis longus and extensor digitorum longus. Find the anterior tibial vessels and deep peroneal nerve between the tibialis anterior and extensor hallucis longus.

In the lateral region of the leg, clean and separate the peroneus longus and brevis. Find the superficial peroneal nerve between those muscles.

In front of the ankle joint, observe the superior and inferior extensor retinacula, cut it longitudinally, trace the muscles attachment along their dissected tendons and the dorsal artery of foot along the tibial artery. Try to find the branches of the dorsal artery of foot—the arcuate artery and deep plantar branch. Trace the deep peroneal nerve and its branches.

Ⅱ. Posterior part of the lower limb

1 Position and incisions

Place the cadaver in prone position. Make the following skin incisions:

● Make a posterior median incision from the mid-point of the two posterior superior iliac spines to the tip of coccyx.

● Make a curve incision from the upper end of aforementioned incision along the iliac crest to the anterior superior iliac spine.

● Make an oblique incision from the tip of the coccyx, downward and laterally along the fold of the buttock skirting the anus.

● Extend the anteriorly made transverse skin incision posteriorly in the knee region and leg.

2 Procedures

2.1 Turn over the skin flap laterally

2.2 Dissect the superficial fascia

Remove the superficial fascia of the gluteal region and the back of the thigh. Try to identify the cutaneous branches of the posterior rami of lumbar and sacral nerves which distribute the gluteal region.

Find the posterior femoral cutaneous nerve descending along the deep surface of deep fascia of the thigh and trace it to the upper margin of the popliteal fossa.

Pick up the small saphenous vein as it passes posterior to the lateral malleolus and trace the vein upward to the popliteal fossa, where it joins the popliteal vein. Isolate the sural nerve which accompanies with the small saphenous vein and pierces the deep fascia near the middle of the posterior aspect of the leg. Trace the sural nerve upward to the point where it is formed by the union of the medial sural cutaneous nerve from the tibial nerve and the communicating branch from the common peroneal nerve.

Carefully remove the superficial fascia while preserving the cutaneous nerve, superficial vessels and the iliotibial tract to expose the deep structures.

2.3 Dissect the deep structures

Carefully define the upper and lower borders of the gluteus maximus. Clean the deep fascia along the borders. Then insert fingers beneath the upper and lower borders of the muscles and separate it from underling structures. Cut the muscle near to its origin and reflect laterally, avoid damaging the posterior femoral cutaneous nerve and the sacrotuberous ligament.

Identify and clean the structures in the suprapiriform foramen, observe their arrangement and observe the relationship between sciatic nerve and piriformis. Cut the sacrotuberous ligament to expose the lesser sciatic foramen. Find the internal pudendal vessels and pudendal nerve which emerges from the infrapiriform foramen and passes through the lesser sciatic foramen to enter the ischiorectal fossa.

Cut the origin of the gluteus medius by a curve incision, turn it downward and laterally to its insertion on the greater trochanter. Clean and follow the deep branches of the superior gluteal vessels and the superior gluteal nerve into the gluteus medius, gluteus minimus and the tensor fasciae latae.

Lift the sciatic nerve and clean it, trace downward to the upper margin of popliteal fossa where it divides into the tibial nerve downward and common peroneal nerve outwards.

Remove the deep fascia of the back of the thigh, avoid injurying the small saphenous vein and the cutaneous nerves. Identify the biceps femoris, semitendinosus, semimembranosus and separate them clearly.

Clean and expose the boundaries of the popliteal fossa. Find the common peroneal nerve along the upper lateral boundary of the fossa. It bypasses the fibular neck into the lower leg and divides into the superficial peroneal nerve and deep peroneal nerves. In the midline, there are the tibial nerve, popliteal vein and popliteal artery from shallow to deep. Try to dissect the branches to knee joint of the popliteal artery.

Remove the deep fascia of the surface of triceps fascia, blunt dissection of medial head and lateral heads of gastrocnemius and soleus, cut the muscle and reflect the muscle downward. Clean the origin of the soleus, then cut the muscle near the tendinous arch and turn it down together with the gastrocnemius. Be careful to the deep structure such as the tibial nerve, branches of posterior tibial artery and plantar muscles.

Lift the popliteal artery, clean its branches of the anterior and posterior tibial artery in the lower part of the fossa. Trace the anterior tibial artery to pierce the interosseous membrane, trace the posterior tibial artery and the accompanying tibial nerve to the medial malleolus. Find their branches.

Clean the muscles of the deep layer, the flexor digitorum longus, flexor pollicis longus and tibialis posterior lie from the medial side to the lateral side.

Observe the flexor retinaculum attachment and cut longitudinally, identify and dissect content of malleolar canal—from anterior backward there are the posterior tibial tendon, flexor digitorum longus tendon, posterior tibial vessels, tibial nerve and the flexor pollicis longus tendon. Finally the posterior tibial artery and tibial nerve are divided into medial and lateral planter arteries and nerves.

Ⅲ. The sole of the foot

1 Incisions

Make a longitudinal mid-line incision on the sole of the foot. Make a transverse incision at the roots of the toes.

2 Procedures

Turn the skin flap and superficial fascia from the mid-line laterally.

2.1 Clean the deep fascia

Note that the intermediate portion of the deep fascia is thick to form the plantar aponeurosis. It is triangular in shape. Define that its apex is attached to the calcaneus and its base divides into five slips towards each toe. Then cut it transversely close to the calcaneus. As the plantar aponeurosis is turned distally, separate it from the underlying muscles, vessels and nerves.

2.2 Dissect the muscles of the first layer

Expose the abductor hallucis and abductor digiti minimi, identify the flexor digitorum brevis between the two abductors. Then cut the flexor digitorum brevis close to the calcaneus and the proximal portion of the abductor hallucis, turn them distally.

Follow the posterior tibial vessels and tibial nerve into the sole and dissect the medial and lateral plantar vessels and nerves.

2.3 Dissect the muscles of the second layer

Identify the quadrates plantae, the tendon of the flexor digitorum longus and the tendon of the flexor hallucis longus. Four delicate lumbricales arise from the tendinous slips. Remove the skin and fascia from the middle toe and clean the tendon. Verify the slip of the tendon of the flexor digitorum longus perforates the tendons of the flexor digitorum brevis and passes to its insertion into the base of the distal phalanx. Then cut the tendon of the flexor digitorum longus distal to the attachment of the quadratus plantae and trun it distally, together with the lumbricales.

2.4 Dissect the muscles of the third layer

Identify the flexor hallucis brevis which cover the first metatarsal bone and is comprised of the two heads . Note that the tendon of the flexor hallucis longus runs between the two heads. Verify the adductor hallucis consists of a transverse head and an oblique head. Observe the flexor digiti minimi to the fifth digit. Cut the transverse and oblique head of the adductor hallucis near its origin, turn it toward its insertion.

2. 5 Observe the muscles of the fourth layer

Identify the deep plantar arch and its branches. Observe the seven interosseous muscles between the metatarsal bones. Trace the tendons of the tibialis posterior and peroneus longus to their insertion distally.

Section 3

Clinical application

I. Varicosis of great saphenous vein

Women are more likely to suffer this disease than men, and most patients age from 30 to 70. Injured vein shows elongation, expansion and winding buckling. The disease progresses in long-term standing work and manual labor, such as teacher, barber, surgeon, etc.

II. Femoral hernia

The incidence of femoral hernia is about $3\% \sim 5\%$ out of abdominal external hernia, more common in women over 40 years old. Hernia blocks are often not big and usually a half spherical projection occurs below the inguinal ligament. Hernia content more often is the small intestine and great omentum. The femoral ring itself is small and the around ligaments are tough and firm, so the incarcerated and strangulated hernia easily occurs. Pregnancy is the main reason for the increase of intraabdominal pressure. Increased intraabdominal pressure and relaxed femoral ring cause femoral hernia.

III. Sciatica

There are many causes of sciatica such as the lumbar intervertebral disc prolapse, piriformis syndrome, stenosis of vertebral canal, tumor and other ailments. Among these causes, lumbar disc herniation is the most common cause.

IV. Deep abscess

In the gluteal region, the loose connective tissue around the nerves and vessels is abundant and the deep fascia is thick and compact, so that the deep abscess of this region is usually localized or extends. It might go

1) Through the greater sciatic foramen into the pelvis;

2) Through the lesser sciatic foramen into the ischioanal fossa;

3) Along the sciatic nerve into the popliteal fossa.

V. Knee joint

The knee joint is the most complex and biggest joint in the body. The meniscus injury is common (especially the medial meniscus). Meniscus tear usually needs surgical resection due to poor bloodsupply, but recently some orthopedists advocate reserving the injured meniscus by suture in young patients. After the meniscectomy, the regeneration of hyaline meniscus occurs from the vascular fibroareolar tissue around the periphery of the joint cavity.

VI. Femoral neck fracture

It is a fracture between the femoral head and the base of the femoral neck. It is a very common fracture in the elderly. Nonunion rate ranges from 20% to 30%. Stress fracture of the femoral neck is uncommon, it happened in active individuals with unaccustomed strenuous activity or changes in activity, such as runners or endurance athletes. The blood- supply blocks after fracture and the incidence of femoral head necrosis is about 75%.

VII. Ankle sprain

It is one of the most common joint sprain. Sprain of ankle joint, especially the damage caused by inversion injury, tear or rupture of lateral collateral ligament. When walking, sprinting or high falling, the lateral part of the feet touches the ground suddenly which can tear the ligament and also combine with the lateral melleolus avulsion fracture.

Section 4

Ask yourself

1. Where is the proper site for intramuscular injection at the gluteus area? And why? Where and how the abscess caused by injection diffuse?

2. Where does the femoral hernia always occur? How to identify the inguinal hernia?

3. Where does the lower end tend to displace in the lower one third of femur shaft fracture? And why is that? What structural damage might be cause?

4. What deformations might result when the lower leg muscles paralysis?

5. Please explain the surface markings of the femoral artery, dorsal artery of foot and sciatic nerve.

6. What are the structures passing through the suprapiriform foramen and infrapiriform, respectively?

7. Describe the boundary and contents of the femoral triangle, the popliteal fossa and the malleolar canal.

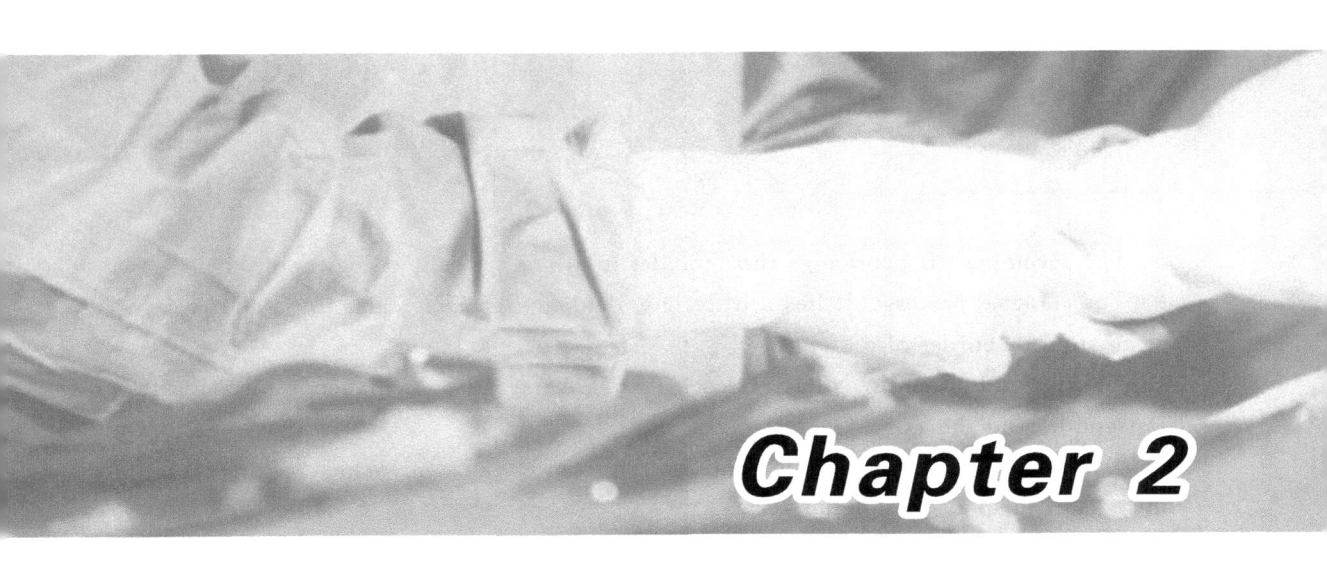

Chapter 2

The upper limb

Section 1

Review

Ⅰ. Surface anatomy

The **acromion** It overhangs the shoulder joint and is easily recognizable.

The **coracoid process** It lies a little lateral to the infraclavicular fossa and is covered by the anterior border of deltoid.

Anterior and posterior axillary folds They are the musculocutaneous folds located in front and behind the axilia respectively .

Biceps brachii It is the prominence on the front of the arm. When the muscle is fully contracted it displays a globular form.

The **deltoid tuberosity** It appears on the lateral surface of the middle third of the humerus. The deltoid is inserted into it.

The **medial and lateral epicondyles of humerus** They are palpable easily and important in the diagnosis of elbow injury.

The **olecranon of ulna** It can always be identified at the back of the elbow joint. When the forearm is fully flexed, the olecranon and the epicondyles form the angles of an equilateral triangle. When the forearm is extended fully,the olecranon and the epicondyles lie in the same horizontal plane.

The **head of radius** It can be touched under the lateral epicondyle of humerus.

The **tendon of biceps brachii** It could be touched in the anterior cubital region, especially half flexion of elbow.

The **styloid process of radius and ulna** They are the ulnar and radial processes of the wrist, respectively.

The **crease of wrist** There are three creases of wrist. The proximal crease of wrist is located in the level of the head of ulna. The middle crease of wrist is not always constant. The distal crease of wrist is situated in the level of the proximal edge of the flexor retinaculum.

The **anatomical snuffbox** The anatomical snuffbox is a superficial pit which located in the lateral part of the dorsum of hand. Its radial boundary is the tendon of abductor pollicis longus and tendon of extensor pollicis brevis. Its ulnar boundary is the tendon of extensor pollicis longus. Its proximal boundary is styloid process of radius. Its fundus is the scaphoid bone and trapezium bone. The radial artery situates in the anatomical snuffbox and can be touched its pulse.

II. Boundaries and divisions

The boundary between upper limb and the neck is the line between the lateral-middle part of the upper edge of clavicle, acromion and the spinous process of the 7th cervical vertebra. The boundary with the thorax is the line between the upper part of the anterior edge of the deltoid and the middle point of the lower edge of the anterior axillary fold. The boundary with the back is the line between the upper part of the posterior edge of the deltoid and the middle point of the lower edge of the posterior axillary fold.

The upper limb is divided into the shoulder, the arm, the elbow, the forearm, the wrist and the hand. The shoulder is subdivided into axilla, the scapular region and the pectoral region. The hand is subdivided into palm, the dorsum and the fingers.

III. Main contents

1 Axillary fossa

1.1 Composition

It comprises one apex, one base and four walls.

● Apex   The apex is surrounded by the middle part of clavicle, the lateral edge of the 1st rib and upper edge of the scapula.

● Base   The base is composed of the skin, superficial fascia and axillary fascia.

● Four   They include the anterior and posterior walls, medial and lateral walls.

The anterior wall is composed of the pectoralis major, pectoralis minor, subclavius and clavipectoral fascia. The cephalic vein, thoracoacromial vessels and lateral pectoral nerve traverse the clavipectoral fascia.

The posterior wall is composed of latissimus dorsi, teres major, subscapularis and scapula. There are trilateral foramen and quadrilateral foramen on the posterior wall. The circumflex scapular vessels pass through the trilateral foramen. The axillary nerve and posterior humeral circumflex vessels traverse the quadrilateral foramen.

The medial wall is composed of serratus anterior, the 1st – 4th ribs and intercostal muscles.

The lateral wall is composed of coracobrachialis, two heads of biceps brachii, intertubercular sulcus of the humerus.

1. 2 Contents

1.2.1 Axillary artery

Axillary artery is divided into three parts by the pectoralis minor.

The first part gives off one branch—the superior thoracic artery, which distributes the front of the 1st and 2nd intercostal space.

The second part has two branches which are thoracoacromial artery and lateral thoracic artery. The thoracoacromial artery traverses the clavipectoral fascia and distributes the pectoralis major and minor, deltoid and acromion. The lateral thoracic artery distributes serratus anterior, pectoralis major and minor and breast.

The third part can be divided into three branches, which are subscapular artery, anterior and posterior humeral circumflex arteries. Subscapular artery is divided into circumflex scapular artery and thoracodosal artery. The former traverses trilateral foramen to infraspinous fossa. The later which concomitant thoracodosal nerve distributes in latissimus dorsi. Posterior humeral circumflex artery traverses quadrilateral foramen from anterior to posterior and anastomose with anterior humeral circumflex artery.

1.2.2 Axillary vein

Axillary vein is lacated at the medial side of axillary artery.

1.2.3 Brachial plexus

The subclavian part of brachial plexus is composed of three cords. The lateral cord gives off the lateral pectoral nerve and musculocutaneous nerve. The medial cord gives off the medial pectoral nerve, medial antebrachial cutaneous nerve, medial brachial cutaneous nerve and ulnar nerve. The medial and lateral roots of median nerve branch from the medial cord and lateral cord, respectively. The posterior cord gives off the radial nerve, axillary nerve, subscapular nerve and thoracodorsal nerve. In addition, the long thoracic nerve originates from supraclavicular part of brachial plexus and innervates serratus anterior.

1.2.4 Axillary lymph nodes

Axillary lymph nodes can be divided into five groups.

● Lateral lymph nodes   They arrange along the distal extremity of axillary vein, and receive the superficial and deep lymphatic vessels of the upper limb. Its efferent lymphatic vessels drain into central lymph nodes.

● Pectoral lymph nodes   They arrange along lateral thoracic vessels, and receive the lymphatic vessels of thoracic antero-external wall, abdominal wall above the umbilicus, the lateral and central parts of breast. Its efferent lymphatic vessels drain into central lymph nodes.

● Subscapular lymph nodes   They arrange along subscapular vessels, and receive the lymphatic vessels of scapular region, thoracic posterior wall and the back. Its efferent lymphatic vessels drain into central lymph nodes too.

● Central lymph nodes　They are located in the adipose tissue of bottom of axillary fossa, and receive the lymphatic vessels of the abovementioned three groups. Its efferent lymphatic vessels drain into apical lymph nodes.

● Apical lymph nodes　They arrange along the proximal extremity of axillary vein and receive the efferent lymphatic vessels of the central lymph nodes. Its most efferent lymphatic vessels converge into subclavian trunk, and the others drain into supraclavicular lymph nodes.

1.2.5　Axillary sheath

It is a fascial sheath which the deep layer of the deep cervical fascia extends and forms in the axillary fossa, it encloses the axillary artery and vein, subclavian brachial plexus.

2　Arm

2.1　Anterior brachial region

2.1.1　Superficial structures

● Skin and superficial fascia　The skin is thin and elastic, while the superficial fascia is thin and loose.

● Superficial veins　Including the cephalic vein and basilic vein.

The cephalic vein originates from the radial part of dorsal venous rete of hand, ascends and traverses clavipectoral fascia to drains into the axillary vein or the subclavian vein.

The basilic vein originates from the ulnar part of dorsal venous rete of hand, traverses the brachial fascia and drains into brachial vein or the axillary vein.

● Cutaneous nerve　It contains the superior lateral brachial cutaneous nerve and inferior lateral brachial cutaneous nerve, the intercostobrachial nerve and medial brachial cutaneous nerve. The medial antebrachial cutaneous nerve is concomitant with basilic vein to the medial side of forearm.

2.1.2　Deep structures

● Deep fascia and osseofascial compartment　The deep fascia of the arm is called the brachial fascia. The brachial fascia ascends and changes into the deltoid fascia, pectoral fascia, and axillary fascia, and descends to the antecubital fascia. The brachial fascia sends out the medial and lateral intermuscular septa. The medial and lateral intermuscular septa, the deep fascia and humerus compose the osseofascial compartment.

● Anterior group of brachial muscle　Including biceps brachii, coracobrachialis, and brachialis.

● Brachial artery　The brachial artery extends from the axillary artery. At the level of the neck of radius, it divides into the radial and ulnar arteries. The branches of brachial artery including:

The deep brachial artery descends into the humeromuscular tunnel, and supplies the triceps brachii.

The superior ulnar collateral artery traverses the medial intermuscular septum with ulnar nerve, and reaches the posterior brachial region.

Inferior ulnar collateral artery.

● Brachial veins   There are two brachial veins accompanying with the brachial artery.

● Nerves

The median nerve is formed by the lateral and medial root, it descends in the medial sulcus of the biceps brachii with the brachial vessels.

The ulnar nerve originates from the medial cord of brachial plexus, it lies in the medial side of brachial artery at the upper part of arm.

The radial nerve begins from the posterior cord of brachial plexus, it lies in the posterior of brachial artery at the upper part of arm.

The musculocutaneous nerve originates from the lateral cord. It's terminal branch emerges between biceps brachii and brachialis at the superolateral of the cubital fossa, it becomes the lateral antebrachial cutaneous nerve.

2.2   Posterior brachial region

2.2.1   Superficial structures

● Skin and superficial fascia   The skin of posterior brachial region is thicker than the anterior brachial region. The superficial fascia is denser than anterior.

● Superficial veins   The superficial veins are small.

● Cutaneous nerves   Including: the superior lateral brachial cutaneous nerve, the inferior lateral brachial cutaneous nerve and the posterior brachial cutaneous nerve.

2.2.2   Deep structures

● Deep fascia and posterior osseofascial compartment of arm   The deep fascia is thick in the posterior brachial region. The deep fascia, medial and lateral intermuscular septa, and humerus form the posterior osseofascial compartment of arm.

● Humeromuscular tunnel   It is formed by the triceps brachii and sulcus for radial nerve, through which the radial nerve and deep brachial vessels pass.

The radial nerve originates from the posterior cord of brachial plexus. The muscular branch of radial nerve innervates triceps brachii.

The deep brachial artery passes through the humeromuscular tunnel where it divides into the radial collateral artery and middle collateral branch.

The deep brachial veins locate at the two sides of deep brachial artery.

3 Elbow

3.1 Anterior cubital region

3.1.1 Superficial structures

● Skin and superficial fascia   The skin is thin and soft, while the superficial fascia is loose.

● Superficial veins   The cephalic vein and basilic vein are located in the lateral and medial side of the biceps tendon respectively.

● Cutaneous nerve   Includes the medial and laternal lutebrachial cutaneous nerve. The medial antebrachial cutaneous nerve accompanies the basilic vein. The lateral antebrachial cutaneous nerve accompanies the cephalic vein at posteromedial side.

● Superficial cubital lymph nodes   They are also called supratrochlear lymph nodes which lies in just above the medial epicondyle of humerus, and are adjacent to the basilic vein. They receive they the superficial lymphatic vessel of the hand and forearm in the ulnar half.

3.1.2 Deep structures

● Boundaries   The superior boundary is the imagary line between the medial and lateral epicondyle of humerus. The inferolateral boundary is the brachioradialis. The inferomedial boundary is the pronator teres.

● Contents   From the ulnar to radial, these structures include the median nerve, brachial artery and its two accompanying veins, biceps tendon, radial nerve and its branches.

3.2 Posterior cubital region

The major structures of posterior cubital region contains tendon of triceps brachii, vessels and ulnar nerve.

4 Forearm

4.1 Anterior antebrachial region

4.1.1 Superficial structures

● Superficial structures   The skin of the anterior antebrachial region is thin and mobility.

● Superficial veins

Cephalic vein is located in radial forearm, then turns anteriorly at the half upper part of forearm.

The basilic vein is located in ulnar forearm, it turns anteriorly inferior to the cubital fossa.

The median antebrachial vein usually joins the median cubital vein or the basilic vein.

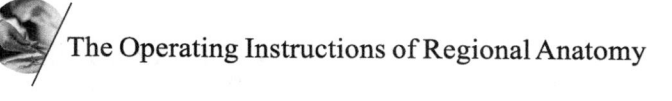

● Cutaneous nerves

The lateral antebrachial cutaneous nerve spreads over the lateral skin of the forearm.

The medial antebrachial cutaneous nerve innervates the medial skin of anterior forearm and the medial skin of posterior forearm, respectively.

4.1.2　Deep Structures

● Deep fascia　The deep fascia of the anterior antebrachial region is thin but flexible.

● Anterior antebrachial osseofascial sheath

Formation—it is surrounded by the deep fascia, the medial and lateral antebrachial intermuscular septa, radius, ulna and the interosseous membrane of forearm.

Contents—there are the anterior muscle groups of forearm, the radial and ulnar neurovascular bundle, the anterior interosseous nerves and vessels and the median nerve.

● Four neurovascular bundles

The radial neurovascular bundle consists of radial artery, the concomitant vein and the superficial branch of radial nerve.

The ulnar neurovascular bundle includes ulnar artery, ulnar vein and ulnar nerve.

The median neurovascular bundle consists of median nerve and concomitant vessels.

The anterior interosseous neurovascular bundle consists of the anterior interosseous nerve and anterior interosseous vessels.

4.2　Posterior antebrachial region

4.2.1　Superficial structures

● Skin　The skin of the posterior antebrachial region is thicker and denser than the anterior antebrachial region.

● Cutaneous nerves　The posterior cutaneous nerve of forearm supply the middle part skin of the back of the forearm, the medial and lateral antebrachial cutaneous nerve supply to the medial and lateral part skin of the back of the forearm.

4.2.2　Deep structures

● Deep fascia　It is thick and strong. In the posterior antebrachial osseofascial sheath, there are the posterior muscles of the forearm and the posterior interosseous neurovascular bundle.

● Posterior interosseous neurovascular bundle　It consists of fine posterior interosseous vessels and nerves, and it locates between the superficial layer and deep layer posterior muscles of the forearm.

5　Wrist

5.1　Anterior region

5.1.1　Superficial structures

The skin of anterior region is thin and loose, and usually forms three creases (refer Chapter 2 Section 1: I. Surface Anatomy). It is innervated by the branches of the medial and lateral antebrachial cutaneous nerve.

5.1.2　Deep structures

● Palmar carpal ligament　It can anchor, protect and support the forearm flexor tendons.

● Flexor retinaculum　It is also called the transverse carpal ligament. Its ulnar end is attached to the pisiform and the hook of hamate. Its radial end is attached to the tubercles of scaphoid and trapezium.

● Ulnar carpal canal　Ulnar carpal canal is a space between flexor retinaculum and palmar carpal ligament, which contains ulnar artery, ulnar vein and ulnar nerve.

● Carpal canal　It is formed by the flexor retinaculum and the groove of carpal bones. It includes the tendons of flexor digitorum superficialis, flexor digitorum profundus enclosed in common flexor sheath, tendon and tendinous sheath of flexor pollicis longus and median nerve.

The common flexor sheath forms the ulnar capsule and the tendinous sheath of flexor pollicis longus forms the radial capsule.

● Radial carpal canal　The radial end of flexor retinaculum is divided into two layers attaching to the tubercles of scaphoid and trapezium, respectively. Radial carpal canal is located between the two layers, where tendon and tendinous sheath of the flexor carpi radialis pass.

5.2　Posterior carpal region

5.2.1　Superficial structures

The skin of posterior region of wrist is thinner than anterior region.

5.2.2　Deep structures

● Extensor retinaculum　The deep fascia of posterior region of wrist is thickened and forms the extensor retinaculum (the dorsal carpal ligament).

● Carpal extensor tendon and tendinous sheaths　They arrange from the radial side to the ulnar side and pass through each osseofibrous canals as follows: ① the tendon and tendinous sheath of abductor pollicis longus and extensor pollicis brevis; ② the tendon and tendinous sheath of the extensor carpi radialis longus and brevis; ③ the tendon and tendinous sheath of extensor pollicis longus; ④ the tendon and tendinous sheath of extensor digitorum and extensor indicis; ⑤ the tendon and tendinous sheath of extensor digiti mini-mi and the tendon and tendinous sheath of extensor carpi ulnaris.

6　The palm of hand

6.1　Layers of the palm

From shallow to deep: skin; the superficial fascia; the superficial layer of deep fascia (palmar aponeurosis, thenar fascia and hypothenar fascia); superficial palmar arch, median nerve, superficial branches of ulnar nerve; the deep layer of deep fascia, muscles and tendons; deep palmar arch and deep branches of ulnar nerve; interosseous muscles and metacarpal bone.

6.1.1　Skin

The Skin is thick, tight and low elasticity.

6.1.2　Superficial fascia

It is loose, but the center of palm is dense and connects with the palmar aponeurosis.

6.1.3　Superficial layer of deep fascia

● Palmar aponeurosis　It is formed by diffuse tendinous fibers of tendon of palmaris longus and thickened. Its shape is a triangular. The distal part of palmar aponeurosis is divided into four longitudinal fibrous bundles which runs to the bottom of the 2nd~5th pha-langette.

● Thenar fascia and hypothenar fascia　They are thin which cover the thenar muscles and the hypothenar muscles, respectively.

6.1.4　Superficial palmar arch, median nerve and superficial branches of ulnar nerve

● Superficial palmar arch　It is formed by the superficial palmar branch of radial artery and the end of ulnar artery. It gives off three common palmar digital arteries which run along with the superficial surface of the 2nd~4th lumbricales to the web's space. Each common palmar digital artery is divided into two proper palmar digital arteries which supply the adjacent sides of the proximal finger. The common palmar digital arteries anasto-mose with palmar metacarpal arteries of deep palmar arch.

● Median nerve　It gives off a recurrent branch and three common palmar digital nerves. Each of common palmar digital nerves divides into two proper palmar digital nerves.

● Superficial branches of ulnar nerve　They give off a proper digital nerve and a common palmar digital nerve, which is divided into two proper palmar digital nerves for the skin of 4th and 5th fingers. The proper digital nerve innervates the skin of ulnar side of the little finger.

6.1.5　Deep layer of the deep fascia, muscles and tendons

● Deep layer of deep fascia of palm　It contains the palmar interosseous fascia and the fascia of adductor pollicis. The deep one is thinner than the superficial layer.

● **Muscles** The muscles of hand can be divided into three groups: the lateral group, the medial group and the intermediate group.

6.1.6 Deep palmar arch and deep branch of ulnar nerve

● Deep palmar arch It is formed by the terminal part of radial artery and the deep palmar branch of ulnar artery. The convexity of deep palmar arch branches three palmar metacarpal arteries which anastomose with the corresponding common palmar digital arteries at metacarpophalangeal joints respectively.

● Deep branch of ulnar nerve It is thinner than the superficial branch and contains motor fibres. Deep branch is concomitant with the deep palmar branch of ulnar artery. It gives off branches to supply the all muscles of hypothenar, the seven interosseus, the 3rd and 4th lumbricals and adductor pollicis.

6.1.7 The interosseous muscles and metacarpal bone

There are three palmar interossei and four dorsal interossei.

6.2 Osseofascial compartments

There are three osseofascial compartments in the palm, the lateral, intermediate and medial osseofascial compartment.

● Lateral osseofascial compartment It is also call the thenar compartment. It is enclosed by the thenar fascia, the lateral intermuscular septum of palm and the 1st metacarpal. It contains abductor pollicis brevis, flexor pollicis brevis, opponens pollicis, the tendon and tendinous sheath of the flexor pollicis longus and vessels and nerves of thumb.

● Intermediate osseofascial compartment It is also known as the palmar central compartment. It is enclosed by the palmar aponeurosis, the lateral intermuscular septum of palm, the medial intermuscular septum of palm, the palmar interosseous fasciae and the fasciae of adductor pollicis. It contains the flexor tendons and their common sheath of digitorum superficialis and profundus, lumbricalis, superficial palmar arches, vessels and nerves of the finger.

● Medial osseofascial compartment It is also called the hypothenar compartment which enclosed by the hypothenar fascia, the medial intermuscular septum of palm and the 5th metacarpal. It contains abductor digiti minimi, flexor digiti minimi brevis, opponens digiti minimi and vessels and nerves of little finger.

6.3 Fascial space

Fascial space is located in the deep of intermediate compartment of palm. There are two fascial spaces.

● Midpalmar space It is located under the ulnar side of palmar intermediate compartment. Midpalmar space extends distally along with the 2nd~4th lumbrical canals and communicates with the 2nd~4th web's spaces to opisthenar. Midpalmar space extends proximally to the deep of common flexor sheath, and communicates with the deep space of forearm flexor muscle through carpal canal.

● Thenar space   It is located under the radial side of palmar intermediate compartment. Thenar space is blind at the proximal end and extends distally to the 1st lumbrical canal. It communicates with the back of index finger.

7   The dorsum of hand

7. 1   Layers of the dorsum of hand

From shallow to deep: skin; the superficial fascia (there are dorsal venous rete of hand, superficial lymphatics and cutaneous nerve in the superficial fascia); the deep fascia (dorsal aponeurosis, dorsal interosseous fascia); tendons of extensor digitorum; interosseous muscles and metacarpal bone.

7. 2   Fascia space

There are two fascia spaces among the superficial fascia, dorsal aponeurosis of hand and dorsal interosseous fascia. The two spaces connect with each other.

● Dorsal subcutaneous space   It is the space between the superficial fascia and dorsal aponeurosis of hand.

● Subaponeurotic space   It is the space between dorsal aponeurosis of hand and dorsal interosseous fascia.

Section 2

Dissection and observation

1 Position and incisions

The cadaver is placed supinely, and the bony landmarks on the cadaver should be palpated before making the skin incision, they are: the jugular notch, sternum, clavicle, and acromion, etc. The incisions should be shallow to avoid damaging deep structures. Detailed incisions should be made as follows:

● Make a median incision at anterior thoracic region from jugular notch to the xiphoid process along the anterior median line.

● Make a superior incision from jugular notch to the acromion along the clavicle.

● Make an inferior incision from the xiphoid process to the posterior axillary line along the costal arch.

● Make an oblique incision from the xiphoid process to the areola of breast, around the nipple to the upper part of the anterior axillary fold, then downward to the upper-middle part of arm along medial border of the arm. Finally, make a horizontal circular incision at the upper-middle part of arm.

Turn the flaps from the medial side to lateral.

2 Procedures

2.1 Dissection of superficial structures

2.1.1 Dissect the female breast

Remove fat on the surface of the mammary gland to expose the outline of lobular of mammary gland. Dissect the lactiferous ducts in the areole carefully with the tip of a blade along the radial direction from nipple and trace the ducts to the lobular of mammary gland. Observe the lactiferous ducts near the nipple.

2.1.2 Dissect the anterior cutaneous branches of intercostal nerves

To identify the 2-7 anterior cutaneous branches of intercostal nerve and the perforating branches of internal thoracic artery at about 1-2 cm lateral of sternum, then cut off the superficial fascia. It would be enough to distinguish two or three branches.

2.1.3   Dissect the supraclavicular cutaneous nerves

Separate and look for the terminal branches of supraclavicular cutaneous nerves below the clavicle.

2.1.4   Dissect the cephalic vein

To identify the intermuscular groove between the deltoid and pectoralis major, and find the cephalic vein from here. 2-3 lymph nodes can be found along the terminal part of the cephalic vein.

2.1.5   Dissect the lateral cutaneous branches of intercostal nerves

Longitudinally cut the superficial fascia along the midaxillary line and the rear of inferior border of pectoralis major. Turn the fascia forward and find the lateral cutaneous branches of intercostal. Intercostobrachial nerve that come from the lateral cutaneous branch of the 2nd intercostal nerve can be seen to go laterally and supply the skin of the upper medial part of arm.

2.2   Dissection of deep structures

2.2.1   Observe the anterior thoracic fascia and the axillary fascia

Remove all of the superficial fascia to expose the deep fascia of the anterolateral thoracic wall. The deep fascia of anterolateral thoracic wall includes a superficial layer and a deep layer. The superficial layer covers the pectoralis major and the serratus anterior. The deep layer envelopes the pectoralis minor and merges with the superficial one at the inferior border of pectoralis minor, finally it connects with the axillary fascia at the bottom of axillary fossa. The deep layer also extends from the superior border of pectoralis minor to the inferior border of clavicle, and forms the clavipectoral fascia that envelops the subclavius just beneath the clavicle.

2.2.2   Expose the pectoralis major

Remove all of the fascia on the surface of pectoralis major. Observe the shape, origin, insertion and direction of muscular fibers of the pectoralis major. Clean and observe the upper and lower margin of the pectoralis major, insert your fingers beneath the muscle from its upper margins to separate it from the thoracic wall. Cut the pectoralis major along a curve line about 2 cm from its origin. Then raise the muscle laterally to show the pectoralis minor and clavipectoral fascia. When the pectoralis major is raised, the thoracoacromial vessels and the lateral pectoral nerve entering into the deep aspect of the muscle at the superior border of pectoralis minor. Further turn the pectoralis major laterally, the branches of medial pectoral nerve can be found entering the pectoralis major after it pierce the pectoralis minor. Clean and observe these vessels and nerves, sufficiently turn the pectoralis major laterally to its insertion, cut small vessels and nerves if needed.

2.2.3　Observe the clavipectoral fascia

The upper part of clavipectoral fascia attaches to the clavicle, the subclavius, the cora-coid process, lower attaches to the superior border of pectoralis minor. Carefully dissect the clavipectoral fascia, clean the thoracoacromial artery, the lateral pectoral nerve and the cephalic vein traversing the clavipectoral fascia. The clavipectoral fascia bonds with the ax-illary sheath tightly and the axillary vein. Remove the clavipectoral fascia and preserve these structures. Split the axillary sheath, dissect the axillary vessels and branches of bra-chial plexus which enveloped by the axillary sheath.

2.2.4　Dissect the structures at the superior border of pectoralis minor

All vessels and nerves are located above the superior border of pectoralis minor and pass through the clavipectoral fascia.

▶ Dissect the lateral pectoral nerve

Carefully clean and trace the lateral pectoral nerve, observe it and its branches. The lateral pectoral nerve originates from the lateral cord of the brachial plexus, passes the front of axillary artery to the deep of clavipectoral fascia, and then pierce the fascia to sup-ply the pectoralis major.

▶ Dissect the thoracoacromial artery

The artery is a short trunk from axillary artery. It is divided into few branches imme-diately. Clean the thoracoacromial artery and trace it to the origin. Observe its branches and distribution.

▶ Dissect the cephalic vein and the subclavian lymph nodes

Try to find lymph nodes under the clavicle near the terminal of cephalic vein. Remove the nodes after observing, then clean the terminal part of the cephalic vein.

2.2.5　Dissect the structures at the surface and inferior border of the pectoralis minor

Clean the fascia on the surface of pectoralis minor and observe the muscle's shape, ori-gin and insertion. The medial pectoral nerve pierces the pectoralis minor and enters the pectoralis major. Cut the pectoralis minor near its origin and turn it upward to coracoid process. After turning over the pectoralis minor, the anterior wall of the axillary fossa is opened. Fully separate the medial pectoral nerve and accompanying vessels from the pecto-ralis minor and preserve them.

▶ Dissect the lateral thoracic artery

Find the lateral thoracic artery and its accompanying veins at the inferior border of pectoralis minor and the surface of serratus anterior. Clean the lateral thoracic artery and trace it to axillary artery.

▶ Observe the pectoral lymph nodes

This group of nodes arrange along the lateral thoracic vessels. Observe them and remove if needed.

2.2.6   Dissect the vessels and nerves related to the lateral wall of the axillary fossa.

Carefully remove the loose connective tissue near the lateral wall of axillary fossa, the residual axillary sheath and the lymph nodes near vessels.

Abduct the arm, remove the axillary fascia and the loose connective tissue at the bottom of axillary fossa. Find and observe the central lymph nodes. After that, clear away these lymph nodes.

Clean the short head of biceps brachii and the coracobrachialis from coracoid process downward.

Dissect the musculocutaneous nerve that enters the coracobrachialis, median nerve and the lateral root of median nerve at the medial border of coracobrachialis. Observe the lateral cord of the brachial plexus.

Follow the median nerve upward, dissect the medial root of median nerve and the axillary artery located between the medial and lateral roots of the median nerve. Observe the medial cord of the brachial plexus.

Dissect the ulnar nerve which comes from medial cord. Observe M-shaped structure which constituted by the musculocutaneous nerve, median nerve and its two roots and ulnar nerve.

Cut off the tributaries of axillary vein and preserve the main trunk of axillary vein.

Find and clean the medial cutaneous nerve of forearm and the medial cutaneous nerve of arm which comes from the medial cord of the brachial plexus, comparing the thickness of the two nerves.

Reset the pectoralis minor, axillary artery which divided into three parts by pectoralis minor. The first part is superior to pectoralis minor, the second part is behind the muscle and the third part is inferior to it. Dissect six branches of the axillary artery. Simple memorizing method: the first part of the axillary artery gives off one branch (superior thoracic artery), the second part gives off two branches (thoracoacromial artery, lateral thoracic artery) and the third one three branches (subscapular artery, anterior and posterior humeral circumflex arteries).

Find radial nerve behind the axillary artery. The radial nerve comes from posterior cord of brachial plexus and trace it downward to the upper part of arm.

2.2.7   Dissect the structures traversing the trilateral foramen and the quadrilateral foramen on the posterior wall of the axillary fossa

▶ Observe the structures traversing the trilateral foramen

On the surface of subscapularis and teres major, find the subscapular artery and its branches, the thoracodorsal artery and the circumflex scapular artery. Trace the circumflex scapular artery which traverses backward to the trilateral foramen.

▶ Observe the structures traversing the quadrilateral foramen

Identify the axillary nerve and the posterior humeral circumflex artery which arises from the axillary artery, trace them traversing backward to the quadrilateral foramen.

2.2.8 Dissect the thoracodorsal nerve

Dissect the thoracodorsal nerve accompanying the thoracodorsal artery and trace it to the latissimus dorsi.

2.2.9 Dissect the superior and inferior branches of subscapular nerve

At the upper part of posterior wall of axillary fossa, find the superior branch of subscapular nerve which supplies the subscapularis. Behind the subscapular artery, find the inferior branch of subscapular nerve and trace it to the teres major.

2.2.10 Dissect the structures at the inferior border of pectoralis major on the medial wall of axillary fossa

Clear the deep fascia on the surface of serratus anterior, find the branches of lateral thoracic vessels at the inferior border of pectoralis major. Behind the lateral thoracic vessels, find the long thoracic nerve along the midaxillary line and trace it upward as far as possible and downward to the serratus anterior. Observe the long thoracic nerve descending to the surface of serratus anterior and supplying it.

Anterior regions of arm, elbow and forearm

1 Position and incisions

The cadaver is placed supinely. Lay the upper limb at abduction position. The skin incision should be shallow and the detailed incisions should be made as follows:

● Make a transverse incision at the midpoint of arm, horizontally, from medial side to the lateral side.

● Make a transverse incision from medial epicondyle of humerus to the lateral epicondyle of humerus.

● The incision is made at the distal wrist crease and extends to the medial and the lateral border of the wrist.

● The incision is made on the anterior aspect of the upper limb from the midpoint of first transverse incision to the second transverse incision, sequentially to the third one.

Turn the skin flap laterally.

2   Procedures

2.1   Dissect the superficial structures

2.1.1   Find the cephalic vein and the lateral cutaneous nerve of the forearm

Trace the cephalic vein downward from deltopectoral groove and clear it up to the wrist. Preserve the cephalic vein and remove the superficial fascia on the anterior region of the arm. In the front of the elbow and the lateral side of the tendon of biceps brachii, find the lateral cutaneous nerve of forearm which pierces the deep fascia and trace it downward to the anterior region of the wrist. Finally, observe the concomitant relation between the lateral cutaneous nerve of the forearm and the cephalic vein.

2.1.2   Dissect the medial cutaneous nerve of the arm

Trace the medial cutaneous nerve of arm which has been dissected downward, the medial cutaneous nerve runs through the fascia and distributes at the skin of medial arm.

2.1.3   Identify the basilic vein and the medial cutaneous nerve of the forearm

Find the basilic vein in the superficial fascia of the lower-middle part of the medial bicipital sulcus. Trace it upward to the middle point of arm in which the basilic vein traverses the deep fascia to brachial vein, and downward to the anterior region of wrist. At the medial region of the upper part of arm, find the medial cutaneous nerve of forearm which has been dissected at the axillary fossa and trace it downward. The medial cutaneous nerve of the forearm may come out through the deep fascia at the lower middle part of the arm and accompanies the basilic vein to the anterior region of wrist.

2.1.4   Dissect the median cubital vein

In the superficial fascia of anterior cubital region, find the median cubital vein which connects the cephalic vein and the basilic vein, observe the connective pattern. It can be cleaned if needed.

2.1.5   Find the cubital lymph nodes

Find the superficial cubital lymph nodes in the upper part of medial epicondyle of humerus and near the basilic vein. These nodes can be cleared after observation.

2.2   Dissect the deep fascia of arm

Remove the superficial fascia at the anterior region of the arm to expose the deep fascia, preserve the superficial veins and the cutaneous nerves that have been dissected out. From the upper arm, longitudinally incise the deep fascia along its middle line and transversely incise at the anterior cubital region. Turn the deep fascia of arm laterally, observe position and attachments of the medial and lateral intermuscular septa of the arm formed by the deep fascia. Finally, clean and observe the muscles of the arm.

2.3 Dissect the medial and lateral bicipital sulci and related vessels and nerves

2.3.1 Dissect the median nerve

From the axillary fossa, trace the median nerve along the medial bicipital sulcus and observe its positional relationship with the brachial artery.

2.3.2 Dissect the brachial artery

From inferior border of teres major, dissect the brachial artery and its two accompanying veins downward to the cubital fossa. Observe and preserve the basilic vein. Cut off the tributaries of brachial vein and preserve its trunk.

2.3.3 Dissect and observe branches of brachial artery

Trace and clean the deep brachial artery which accompanies radial nerve to enter humeromuscular tunnel.

At the level of the insertion of coracobrachialis, find the slender superior ulnar collateral artery and clean. Observe it accompanying the ulnar nerve to pierce the posterior brachial region through the medial brachial intermuscular septum.

At about 5 cm above the medial epicondyle of humerus, look for the inferior ulnar collateral artery and observe its course and position.

Check some muscular branches of the brachial artery and observe their distribution carefully.

2.3.4 Dissect the ulnar nerve

Trace and clean the ulnar nerve downward from the medial cord of brachial plexus to the arm. Observe its positional relationship with the brachial artery and the superior ulnar collateral artery. Dissect the ulnar nerve pierces the medial brachial intermuscular septum to the posterior brachial region.

2.3.5 Dissect structures in lateral bicipital sulcus

Identify the cephalic vein, which has been dissected again, ascending in lateral bicipital sulcus and entering into the deltopectoral groove.

At about 2.5 cm below insertion of deltoid, separate the brachioradialis and the brachialis, and dissociate the radial nerve in the lateral bicipital sulcus. Find the muscular branches of radial nerve, dissect its superficial branch and deep branch in front of lateral epicondyle of humerus. Trace the superficial branch to the deep of brachioradialis and deep branch to supinator, respectively.

2.4 Dissect the cubital fossa

2.4.1 Clear up and identify the borders of the cubital fossa

Find biceps tendon, cut bicipital aponeurosis and deep fascia of cubital fossa at its medial side. Clean the pronator teres and the brachioradialis which form the inferior medial and lateral boundary, respectively. Observe the borders (the superior boundary is an imaginary line connecting medial and lateral epicondyles of the humerus) and the structures on the cubital fossa.

2.4.2 Dissect the structure in the cubital fossa

Biceps tendon and pronator teres as a marker, observe the relationship between the blood vessels and nerves in the cubital fossa. Clean biceps tendon, dissect the brachial artery to its terminal branches, radial and ulnar arteries. Dissect the accompanying veins of brachial artery, clean the median nerve in the medial side of brachial artery and trace it to the two heads of pronator teres. Insert the tip of a hemostatic forceps between the two head of the pronator teres along the trunk of median nerve and cut the humeral origin of it. Examine anterior interosseous nerve at the dorsal part of median nerve. Draw back the ulnar origin of pronator teres and find the ulnar artery and its one branch which called the common interosseous artery at the deep of pronator teres.

2.5 Dissect the deep fascia of forearm, bicipital aponeurosis and palmar carpal ligaments

Remove the superfacial fascia of cubital fossa, anterior regions of the forearm and wrist, preserve the isolated superficial vein and the cutaneous nerves. Show and observe the deep fascia of forearm, then longitudinally incise it to wrist and turn laterally. Probe the medial and the lateral intermuscular septum of forearm and observe their position and attachments. Clean and preserve the bicipital aponeurosis. Observe the deep fascia of anterior carpal region and find transverse fiber thickening part which called the palmar carpal ligaments. Longitudinally incise the radial side of the palmar carpal ligaments to expose the flexor tendons which are deep to it, and the distal flexor retinaculum.

2.6 Dissect the flexor region of the forearm

2.6.1 Observe the superficial layer of anterior group muscles in forearm

Clean up the brachioradialis which originates from the upper part of lateral epicondyle of humerus and the superficial muscles originating from the medial epicondyle of humerus. Then, observe arrangements of each superficial muscle and observe their origins and insertions. Separate the flexor digitorum superficialis from the superficial muscles and observe their tendons.

2.6.2 Dissect the radial vessels and nerve

Pull the brachioradialis laterally and find the radial nerve located between the brachioradialis and the brachialis. Observe the superficial and deep branches of radial nerve. The superficial one descends along the lateral side of radial artery and the deep branch reaches the back of forearm by piercing the supinator. Trace the superficial branch to the low-middle 1/3 of forearm where it is beneath the tendon of brachioradialis and observe it turning to the dorsal part of forearm. Observe the radial artery turning to the opisthenar under the styloid process of radius, observe the branches of the radial artery.

2.6.3   Dissect the ulnar vessels and nerves

Along the midline, cut off the pronator teres and turn to both sides. Pull the flexor carpi ulnaris medially and find the ulnar artery and nerve. Cut off the radial head of the flexor digitorum superficialis at the upper part in the forearm, and turn laterally (Be careful not to damage the median nerve), examine ulnar neurovascular bundle. Trace the ulnar nerve upward to the sulcus for ulnar nerve behind the medial epicondyle of the humerus and downward to the anterior region of wrist, observe its branches supplying the muscles. Observe the relative position between the ulnar nerve and the ulnar artery.

2.6.4   Dissect the median nerve

Find the median nerve that has been dissected between the two heads of pronator teres and trace it to the part between the flexor digitorum superficialis and the flexor digitorum profundus. Clean it to the anterior region of wrist and observe its branches that supply the muscles.

2.6.5   Dissect the deep muscles of the anterior group of forearm

Turn the flexor digitorum superficialis (being cut off) upward, observe the positions and shapes of flexor pollicis longus and flexor digitorum profundus. Separate the two muscles at the upper part of wrist to show the position and shape of pronator quadratus.

2.6.6   Dissect the common interosseous artery and its branches

At the deep of ulnar head of pronator teres, look for the common interosseous artery and clean it. The common interosseous artery gives off an anterior and a posterior interosseous arteries at the upper edge of interosseous membrane of forearm. Find out the anterior interosseous artery and nerve between the flexor pollicis longus and flexor digitorum profundus, trace them upward to the pronator teres and downward to the pronator quadratus. Examine the posterior interosseous artery through the upper edge of interosseous membrane of forearm.

2.6.7   Check the posterior space of the flexor of forearm

Check the posterior space of forearm flexor among flexor pollicis longus, flexor digitorum profundus and pronator quadratus above the wrist. Insert the handle of a knife into the carpal canal and understand its communication with the palm.

Ⅲ. Posterior regions of the arm, elbow and forearm

1 Position and incisions

The cadaver is placed in the prone position with the upper limb abducted. Make incisions as follows:

● Vertical incision on posterior median line of the body: make an incision along the posterior midline from the external occipital protuberance to the spinous process of the 5th lumbar vertebrae.

● Shoulder transverse incision: make an incision from the spinous process of the 7th cervical vertebra to the acromion.

● Through inferior angle of scapula transverse incision: make an incision at the level of inferior angle of scapula, horizontally from the posterior midline to the posterior axillary line.

● Transverse incision at posterior region of arm: make a transverse incision through the midpoint of posterior region of arm, horizontally, from medial side to the lateral side.

● Posterior cubital region transverse incision: make a transverse incision at the posterior cubital region.

● Transverse incision on the dorsum of wrist: make a transverse incision on the back of wrist.

Strip the skin and turn it up to show the superficial fascia.

2 Procedures

2.1 Dissect the superficial layer

Observe the superficial fascia of posterior region of the upper limb, the shoulder superficial fascia is thicker, denser, gradually thinning from the posterior region of the arm to the forearm.

Look for the lateral cutaneous nerve of arm (the cutaneous branches of axillary nerve) in the superficial fascia under the middle of the posterior border of deltoid.

Find out the posterior brachial cutaneous nerve (the cutaneous branches of radial nerve) in the superficial fascia of middle part of posterior brachial region.

Observe the posterior antebrachial cutaneous nerve (the cutaneous branches of radial nerve) at the lateral part of the low-middle 1/3 of posterior brachial region.

Find out the basilic vein, the cephalic vein, the medial and lateral antebrachial cutaneous nerve at the lateral and medial part of the lower part of posterior antebrachial region. Preserve the cutaneous nerves and superficial veins, remove the superficial fascia to expose the deep fascia.

2.2　Dissect deep structures of scapular region

2.2.1　Dissect the suprascapular artery and the suprascapular nerve

Remove the superficial and deep fascia on the surface of trapezius, cut the attachment of trapezius along the spine of scapula. Turn the muscle up and observe the muscles of shoulder behind the scapula.

Cut the supraspinatus and the infraspinatus at the middle part of muscles. Find the suprascapular artery and nerve beneath the muscles.

2.2.2　Dissect the axillary nerve and the posterior humeral circumflex artery

Clean the teres minor, the teres major and the long head of triceps brachii. Examine the boundaries of trilateral and quadrilateral spaces and vessels, nerves which pierce the spaces.

Remove the deep fascia on the surface of deltoid and separate the muscle from the deep structures. Cut the deltoid 1~2 cm away from its origin on the spine of scapula, acromion and clavicle and turn the muscle downward. Observe the axillary nerve and the posterior humeral circumflex artery and vein that pass through the quadrilateral space and supply the deltoid and the teres minor.

2.2.3　Dissect the circumflex scapular artery

Clean the circumflex scapular artery and vein in the trilateral space, and then clean the circumflex scapular artery that leave the space to the infraspinous fossa.

2.3　Dissect deep structures of posterior region of arm

Clean up the deep fascia on the surface of triceps brachii. Make an incision on the deep fascia longitudinally along the middle of posterior arm and turn it two sides to show the triceps brachii.

Obtusely separate the long head of triceps brachii from lateral head to find the humeromuscular canal through which the radial nerve and deep brachial vessels traverse.

Insert the tip of a forceps into the humeromuscular canal along the radial nerve, cut the lateral head of the triceps brachii to open the canal and show the radial nerve and deep brachia artery within the canal. Clean the nerve and artery upward and downward respectively, examine their branches and arrangement pattern.

Find and observe the ulnar nerve, trace it downward to the sulcus of ulnar nerve on humerus.

2.4　Dissect the dorsal deep fascia of forearm and the extensor retinaculum

Preserve the superficial veins and the cutaneous nerves, remove the superficial fascia to show the deep fascia and the extensor retinaculum which thicken from deep fascia on the dorsum of the wrist. Remove the extensor retinaculum and examine the posterior muscles of forearm.

2.5　Dissect the dorsal deep structure of forearm

2.5.1　Dissect the posterior muscles of forearm

Dissect the superficial muscles and observe their shapes, positions, origins and insertions. Separate the extensor carpi radialis brevis from extensor digitorum and laterally to expose supinator. Clean the five deep muscles and check their positions, arrangements, origins and insertions.

2.5.2　Dissect the posterior interosseous vessels and nerves

Find the deep branch of radial nerve in the place where it traverse the supinator. Trace the deep branch downward and find it traversing outward at the middle of supinator and become the posterior interosseous nerve. Clean the posterior interosseous nerve downward to the lower border of supinator. Dissect the posterior interosseous vessels and observe their positions and courses.

Ⅳ. Anterior region of wrist, palm of hand

1　Position and incisions

The cadaver is placed supinely. Detailed incisions should be made as follows.
● Make a longitudinal incision from the middle of the transverse incision of anterior region of wrist to the tip of middle finger.
● Make an oblique incision from the middle of the transverse incision of anterior region of wrist to the tip of thumb.
● Make a transverse incision from the root of the 2nd finger to root of 5th one.
Turn the skin of palmar surface of palm, thumb and middle finger aside.

2　Procedures

2.1　Dissect the superficial fascia

Find the distal branch of lateral cutaneous nerve of forearm, the superficial branch of radial nerve, and the palmar branch of median nerve at the superficial fascia on thenar. Look for the palmar branch of ulnar nerve and observe the palmaris brevis in the fascia on hypothenar. Preserve these cutaneous nerves and remove the superficial fascia to expose the superficial layer of palmar deep fascia.

2.2　Dissect the palmar aponeurosis and osteofascial compartments

2.2.1　Dissect the palmar aponeurosis

Cut off the tendon of palmaris longus above the flexor retinaculum, strip the palmar aponeurosis distally, while cut off the medial and the lateral intermuscular septa of palm, it originate from the medial edge and the lateral edge of palmar aponeurosis, to the interspace of finger web. Cut off palm aponeurosis simutaneously. Turn distally the palmar aponeurosis and protect the structures deep to it.

2.2.2　Examine three osteofascial compartments

The intermediate compartment is located in the deep of palmar aponeurosis, the medial compartment is located in the deep of hypothenar fascia and the lateral one in the deep of thenar fascia. Probe them and remove the hypothenar fascia and the thenar fascia to expose the intrinsic muscle of hand.

2.3　Dissect the ulnar nerve, ulnar artery and their branches

2.3.1　Dissect the ulnar artery and its branches

At the radial part of pisiform bone, cut the palmar carpal ligaments. Open the ulnar carpal canal and clean the ulnar artery and vein in the canal, distally trace the ulnar artery and observe the deep palmar branch which comes from the ulnar artery in the canal. Dissect the superficial palmar arch which formed by the terminal of ulnar artery and the superficial palmar branch of radial artery, and clean the three common palmar digital arteries which originate from the superficial palmar arch to the finger web.

2.3.2　Dissect the ulnar nerve and its branches

In the ulnar carpal canal, clean and observe the ulnar nerve dividing into the superficial branch and the deep branch between the pisiform bone and the hamate bone. Strip the superficial branch downward and observe its branches and arrangement on palm.

2.4　Dissect the median nerve and its branches

2.4.1　Dissect the carpal canal

Clean the flexor retinaculum and longitudinally incise it. Separate the flexor tendon, the flexor tendon sheath and the median nerve passing through the carpal canal.

2.4.2　Clean the median nerve in the carpal canal

Find the recurrent branch of the median nerve at the lower edge of flexor retinaculum and trace it to the thenar muscles. Trace three common palmar digital nerves of median nerve downward to the interspace of finger web, observe their arrangements with the accompanying vessels.

2.5　Examine the flexor tendon sheath

Longitudinally incise the common flexor tendon sheath in the carpal canal and distally probe its relation with the synovial sheaths of fingers. Observe the positional relation between the tendon of flexor digitorum superficialis and the tendon of flexor digitorum profundus. Incise the tendon sheath of flexor pollicis longus and observe its relation with the synovial sheath of thumb.

2.6 Dissect and observe the deep structures of palm

2.6.1 Dissect the thenar muscles

At the medial edge of thenar muscles, find superficial palmar branch of radial artery which anastomoses with the ulnar artery to form the superficial palmar arch, preserve superficial palmar branch of radial artery and recurrent branch of median nerve. Observe the two superficial muscles on thenar. Then cut them on the middle and observe the two deep muscles and the tendon of flexor pollicis longus.

2.6.2 Dissect the hypothenar muscles

Examine the two superficial muscles. Find the deep branch of ulnar nerve and the deep palmar branch of ulnar artery. Transversely cut the abductor digiti minimi and observe the opponens digiti minimi.

2.6.3 Dissect the lumbricals

Separate the tendon of flexor digitorum superficialis and the tendon of flexor disitorum profundus, observe the origin and insertion of lumbricals and its arrangement.

2.6.4 Dissect the interspace of finger web

Remove the fat in the interspaces of finger web. Clean the terminals of each common palmar digital arteries and nerves, observe their branches and distributions. Clean the tendon of lumbricals. Probe the communication of the interspaces of finger web.

2.6.5 Probe the interfascial spaces of palm

Pick up the tendon of forefinger flexor and the first lumbricalis by the hemostatic forceps to observe the deep thenar space. Raise the tendons of the 3rd, 4th and 5th finger flexores and the 2nd, 3rd and 4th lumbricalises to observe the deep midpalmar space and probe proximally its communication with the forearm.

2.6.6 Dissect the deep palmar arch and the deep branch of ulnar nerve

Pull all tendons of finger flexor and lumbricalis to radial side or cut them at the proximal part of carpal canal, and remove the deep loose connective tissue and the palmar interosseous fascia. Trace the deep branch of ulnar nerve and the deep palmar branch of ulnar artery, which have been dissected, to the radial side. Observe the deep palmar arch that is formed by the deep palmar branch of ulnar artery and the terminal of radial artery. Clean the deep palmar arch and its branches at the convex side including three palmar metacarpal arteries. Clean the concomitant deep branch of ulnar nerve and its branches.

2.7 Dissect the palmar structures of fingers

Clean the proper palmar digital nerves and vessels from the interspaces of finger web to the distal end and observe their positions. Remove the superficial fascia to expose the fibrous sheathes at the palmar surfaces of fingers. Longitudinally incise the fibrous sheathes, observe the positional relation between the flexor digitorum superficialis and the flexor disitorum profundus and their insertions. Observe the structure of synovial tendon sheath.

Posterior region of wrist, dorsal aspect

1 Position and incisions

Place the cadaver in the prone position. Follow the instructions to incise.

● Make an oblique incision from the middle of transverse incision of dorsal wrist to the nail root of thumb.

● Make a longitudinal incision from the middle of transverse incision of dorsal wrist to the nail root of middle finger.

● Make longitudinal incisions along the middle line of forefinger, middle finger and ring finger.

● Make a transverse incision along the dorsum of metacarpophalangeal joints, from lateral side of 2nd finger to medial side of 5th finger.

Turn up or cut off the skin of dorsum of hand.

2 Procedures

2.1 Dissect superficial structures of the dorsum of hand

2.1.1 Dissect the superficial fascia of dorsum of hand

Clean, observe and protect the superficial veins and the cutaneous nerves in the dorsum of hand.

2.1.2 Dissect the dorsal venous rete of hand

Observe and clean the dorsal venous rete of hand in the superficial fascia. Examine the cephalic vein at the radial side of the hand and the basilic vein at ulnar side.

2.1.3 Dissect the superficial branch of the radial nerve and the dorsal branch of ulnar nerve

Find the superficial branch of radial nerve at the proximal part of dorsum of the hand and dissect the branch of ulnar nerve at the ulnar side of dorsum. Observe their anastomoses at the dorsum and the arrangement and distribution of the five dorsal digital nerves.

2.1.4 Dissect the six osseofibrous canals formed by the extensor retinaculum and observe the tendons passing though the canals

Remove the superficial fascia of dorsum of wrist to expose the extensor retinaculum, observe the shape and attachment. Longitudinally incise the extensor retinaculum and observe five fibrous compartments beneath it. Clean six tendons and their tendinous sheaths in the six osseofibrous canals and observe each tendon of extensor digitorium and their tendinous sheaths.

2.1.5　Dissect the arteries on dorsum

Clean the three long tendons to thumb at the radial side of the dorsum, and observe the boundaries of the anatomical snuff box. Remove the loose connective tissue in the anatomical snuff box and clean the radial artery and vein in the box. Trace the vessels upward to the anterior region of the forearm and downward to the part where they traverse the first dorsal interossei into palm.

2.2　Dissect the interfascial spaces of dorsum

Preserve the superficial veins and the tegumentary nerve, gradually remove the superficial fascia to show the opisthenar aponeurosis and observe the opisthenar subcutaneous space. Remove the opisthenar aponeurosis to show the interosseous dorsal fascia and observe the opisthenar subaponeurotic space. Observe the intertendinous connections of extensor digitorum.

2.3　Dissect the dorsal surfaces of fingers

Trace the tendons of extensor digitorum to the dorsal surfaces and observe the dorsal aponeurosis on the fingers.

Section 3

Clinical application

I. Deltoid paralysis

The deltoid is innervated by axillary nerve. Axillary nerve passes through the quadrangular space and winds around the surgical neck of the humerus. It can be injured by dislocation of the shoulder joint, fracture of the surgical neck, or long time on crutch. Deltoid paralysis immobilized abduction of shoulder joint. Without timely treatment, it can lead to flattened shoulder as the deltoid atrophy.

II. "Wrist drop"

The posterior group muscles of forearm extend the wrist joint. These muscles are innervated by radial nerve which comes from posterior cord of brachial plexus. Radial nerve descends downward through humeromuscular tunnel along the radial groove of humerus which fracture of the humerus lead to radial nerve injury. Thus, "wrist drop" is resulted.

III. Carpal canal syndrome

Increased pressure of carpal canal syndrome lead to compression of the median nerve. The most common cause of increased pressure in the carpal canal is idiopathic carpal tunnel tendon synovial hyperplasia and fibrosis. The mechanism is still unclear. Common symptoms include sensory abnormalities and / or numbness at the regions (the thumb, index finger, middle finger and ring finger radial side) which are innervated by median nerve, finally the thenar muscles may be paralysed and atrophy.

IV. Winging of the scapula

The long thoracic nerve comes from supraclavicular part of brachial plexus and it innervates serratus anterior. The physiological structure should be preserve as much as possible in radical mastectomy. The lesion of long thoracic nerve may lead to paralysis of ser-

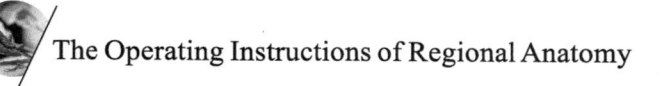

ratus anterior and appears winging of the scapula.

V. "Claw hand"

An claw hand may follow an ulnar nerve lesion which results in the partial or complete denervation of the ulnar two lumbricals of the hand, common injury includes fracture of the medial epicondyle.

It is a deformity or an abnormal attitude of the hand that develops due to ulnar nerve damage causing paralysis of the lumbricals.

Section 4

Ask yourself

1. Describe the contents passing through the trilateral space and the quadrilateral space.

2. Describe the walls and contents of the axilla.

3. What are the boundaries of the cubital fossa? What contents are these in the cubital fossa?

4. Where is the humeromuscular tunnel? What contents are there in it?

5. Describe the structures and formation of carpal canal .

6. What can cause "claw hand"? Why does it happen?

7. Why "ape hand" is displayed when median nerve is injured?

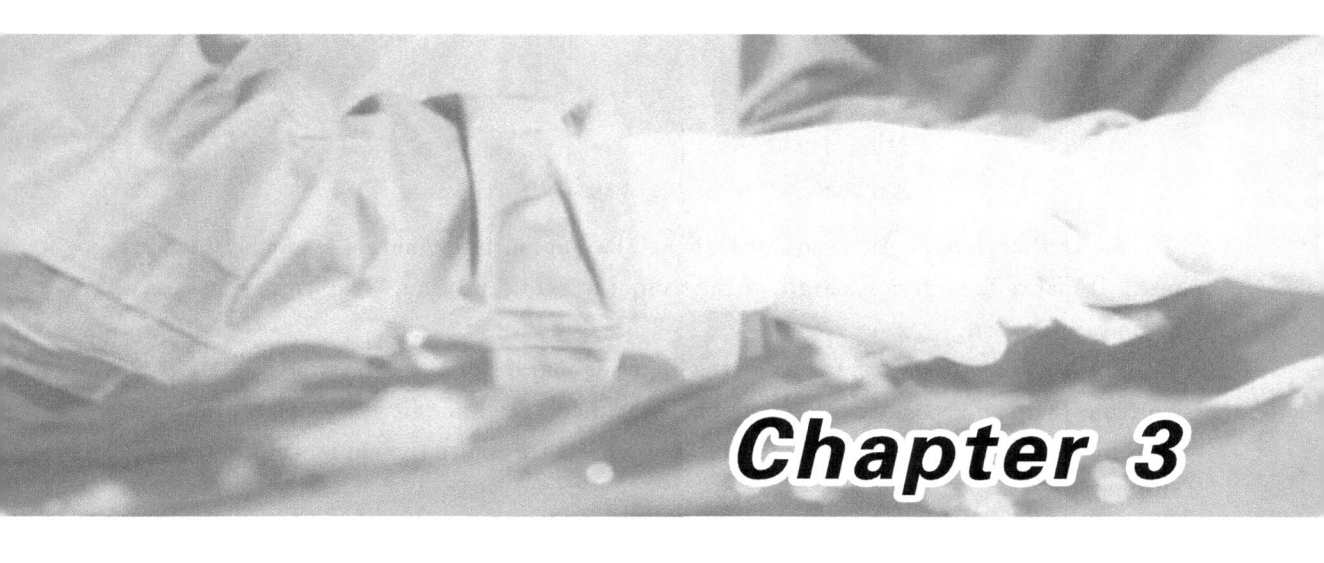

Chapter 3

The head

Section 1

Review

Superciliary arch It is situated above the supraorbital margin which is obvious in men. It marks the inferior margin of the frontal lobe of cerebrum. The frontal sinus is deep to its medial part.

Supraorbital foramen It lies at the superior margin of the orbit which is about 2～3 cm from the median line, or the junction of the medial and middle 1/3 parts of the supraorbital margin. Sometimes it is supraorbital notch. It transmits the supraorbital artery, vein and nerve.

Infraorbital foramen It is located about 0.5～0.8 cm below the infraorbital margin. It transmits the infraorbital vessels and nerve so that it is a point of the blocking anesthesia for the infraorbital nerve.

Mental foramen It lies below the second premolar, and is about 2～3 cm from the median line. At mental foramen, the mental vessels and nerves emerge. Mental foramen is the puncture point for the anesthesia of mental nerve.

The supraorbital foramen, the infraorbital foramen and the mental foramen usually lies on a line.

Pterion Formed by the junction of the sphenoid, frontal, parietal and temporal bones, it is "H" shape which lies about 3.8 cm above the midpoint of the zygomatic arch. It is a feeble site of the cranial bone where the anterior branch of the middle meningeal artery passes through its inner surface. The lateral side of head tends to fracture when hit by force and usually leads to dilaceration of artery and epidural hematoma.

Zygomatic arch It is a bony bridge which located on the horizontal line, it is anterior to the external acoustic pore. Its upper border corresponds to the lower border of the anterior portion of the temporal lobe of the cerebrum. The midpoint of the semilunar area between the inferior margin of the zygomatic arch and the mandibular notch is puncture point for the anesthesia of the maxillary nerve and the mandibular nerve.

Angle of mandible It is the junction of the inferior border of the mandibular body and the posterior margin of the ramus of mandible.

Mastoid process It is a cone-shaped protuberance of the temporal bone which is behind the lower part of the auricle, with the mastoid cells inside. The stylomastoid foramen lies anteromedially to the root of the process and it is the passway of the facial nerve out of the cranium. There is the sulcus for sigmoid sinus on the inner side of the posterior part of the process. The facial nerve and the sigmoid sinus should be protected in radical mastoidectomy.

Bregma It is a rhombus-shaped gap filled with membrane at birth, which called the anterior fontanelle. Usually it will close in the second year.

Lambda It is called posterior fontanelle at birth, which is the junction of the sagittal and lambda sutures.

External occipital protuberance It is a prominence on outer central portion of the squamous part of the occipital bone which is not obvious in children. It corresponds deeply to the sinus confluence and bilaterally to the posterior pole of the occipital lobe of the cerebrum.

Superior nuchal lines They are the ridges which pass laterally from the external occipital protuberance to the mastoid process and corresponds deely to the transverse sinus.

II. Boundaries and divisions

The boundary separating the head from the neck is an imaginary line which linking the lower border of mandible, the angle of mandible, the mastoid process, the superior nuchal line and the external occipital protuberance. The head is divided into two parts: cranium and face.

III. Main contents

1 Cranium

1.1 The fronto-parieto-occipital region

The scalp covers the vertex of the skull and has five layers from superficial to deep.

1.1.1 Skin

It is thick and dense, having hair bulbs, sweat glands and sebaceous glands. It is a frequent region of furuncles and sebaceous cysts. It is liable to bleed and heal due to its abundant blood supply.

1.1.2 Superficial fascia

This layer is mainly composed by dense connective tissue and adipose tissue. Many fibrous bands form numerous pockets where there are vessels and nerve. Those vessels could not contract because its wall is fixed to the fibrous bands. Hemotasis by compression would stop bleeding.

Blood vessels and nerves pass through the lower margin of the scalp to the vertex which can be divided into three groups: the anterior, middle and posterior.

● Anterior group   There are medial and lateral subgroups. The medial subgroup which lies about 2 cm from the median line includes supratrochlear nerve and vessels. The lateral subgroup which lies about 2.5 cm from the median line includes supraorbital nerve and vessels.

● Posterior group   It includes the occipital vessels and greater occipital nerve.

● Lateral group   It can be divided into preauricular group.

1.1.3   Epicranial aponeurosis and occipitofrontalis

It is located at the vertex and is continued with the frontal belly of occipitofrontal anteriorly and occipital belly of occipitofrontalis posteriorly, respectively. Laterally, it becomes thinner and is continued with the temporal fascia. This tough and thick aponeurosis firmly affixes with the skin and the superficial fascia so that these three layers are usually regarded as a single layer (the scalp proper).

Incision of the epicranial aponeurosis, especially transverse injury, should be sutured in case of the wound dehiscence due to contraction of frontal and occipital bellies of the muscle.

1.1.4   The subaponeurotic loose connective tissue

It is a layer of thin, loose connective tissue which is located between the scalp proper and the pericranium. This layer makes the scalp move moderately. It turned to be a dangerous area because infection (blood and pus) can easily spread in this layer or from the scalp to the intracranial sinuses through emissary veins.

1.1.5   Pericranium

It is thin and dense which closely adheres to the sutures of cranial bones. Thus the subpericranial hematoma usually limited within a piece of cranial bone.

1.2   The temporal region

Similarly to the fronto-parieto-occipital region, there are also five layers in the temporal region from superficial to deep.

1.2.1   Skin

It is thin and movable, so it could be sutured easily in operation. The skin scar is hardly visible after repairation.

1.2.2   Superficial fascia

Blood vessels and nerves in this layer can be divided into preauricular group and posterior auricular group.

● Preauricular group   The superficial temporal blood vessels and auriculotemporal nerve emerge at the upper margin of the parotid gland, pass by the zygomatic arch and finally go into the temporal region.

● Posterior auricular group   The posterior auricular vessels and lesser occipital nerve belong to this group and they are distributed in the posterior part of the temporal region.

1.2.3   Temporal fascia

The dense temporal fascia covers the temporalis. Above the zygomatic arch, it is divided into two layers by adipose tissue. The superficial layer is attached to the upper border and outer surface of zygomatic arch. The deep layer is attached to the upper border and inner surface of the arch. There are some adipose tissue and the middle temporal vessels between those two layers.

1.2.4   Temporalis

It is a fan-shaped mastication muscle which originates from the bone surface of temporal fossa and temporal fascia, it passes downward along the deep surface of zygomatic arch and ends at the coronoid process of the mandibular ramus.

1.2.5   Pericranium

It is thin and closely attaches to the surface of the temporal bone. Subpericranial hematoma rarely happened in this region.

2   Superficial part of the face

2.1   The layers of the superficial part

2.1.1   Skin, superficial fascia and, muscles of expression

The skin is rich in blood supply, sebaceous glands, sweat glands and hair follicles which results frequent incidence of furuncle. The muscles of expression situated in the skin and they are supplied by the facial nerve.

2.1.2   Blood supply

The facial artery and homonymous vein are the vessels in the superficial part of the face. The facial artery arises from the external carotid artery in the neck and passes upward by the lower border of the mandible. The facial artery enters into the face at the anterior border of the masseter, then passes along the angle of the mouth, nose, and ends at the medial angle of the eyes. The facial vein runs downward and backward, posterior to the facial artery. It receives the anterior branch of the retromandibular vein before draining into the internal jugular vein.

2.1.3   Nerves

The facial nerve in the superficial part of face and its fan-shaped distrbution branches innervates the muscles of expression. The branches include temporal, zygomatic, buccal, marginal mandibular and cervical branches.

Another nerve in the superficial part of face is the trigeminal nerve which transmits the sense of face skin through its three divisions: ophthalmic nerve, maxillary nerve and mandibular nerve. In addition, the greater auricular nerve supplies the skin over the angle of the mandible and the parotid gland.

2.2 The parotideomasseteric region

2.2.1 Parotid gland

▶ Position

It is an important organ in the parotideomasseteric region. The structures adjacent to the parotid gland are the skin, the superficial fascia (blood vessels and nerves are in it), the parotideomasseteric fascia, the superficial part of parotid gland, the blood vessels and nerves between the superficial part and the deep part of parotid gland, the masseter, the ramus of mandible as well as the deep part of parotid gland from superficial to deep, respectively.

The parotid gland is pyramidal in shape, with its base pointing lateral and its apex medial. It can be divided into the superficial part and the deep part by the posterior border of the mandible or the facial nerve plexus in the parotid gland.

▶ Relations

The parotid region is bounded as follows:

Superiorly—near the zygomatic arch, the external acoustic meatus and the temporomandibular joint.

Inferiorly—at the level of the angle of mandible.

Anteriorly—near the masseter, the ramus of mandible and the posterior border of the medial pterygoid. The superficial part usually extends superficial to the posterior part of the masseter.

Posteriorly—to the anterior border of the mastoid process and the anterior border of the superior part of the sternocleidomastoid.

The deep part of parotid gland is located in the retromandibular fossa and the deep of the ramus of mandible. It is adjacent to the muscles originated from styloid process, internal carotid blood vessels and the last four cranial nerves. Those adjacent structures together form the "bed" of parotid gland.

▶ Sheath

It is formed by the superficial and deep layers of the parotideomasseteric fascia and encloses the parotid gland. The superficial layer of the sheath is dense and thick whereas the deep one is loose and thin.

▶ Parotid duct

It begins from the anterior border of the superficial part of the gland, about 3.5~5 cm long, passes forward by the surface of the masseter, about 1 cm below the zygomatic arch, and then turns medially through the buccal muscle (buccinator), and lastly opens on the mucous membrane opposite to the second upper molar tooth by a papilla. The buccal branch of the facial nerve and the transverse facial vessels accompany with the parotid duct.

The structures passing in the gland are as follows.

The longitudinal group includes the external carotid artery, the superficial temporal vessels, the retromandibular vein and the auriculotemporal nerve.

The transversal group includes the maxillary vessels, the transverse facial vessels and the facial nerve.

From superficial to deep, they are the facial nerve and its branches, the retromandubular vein, the external carotid artery and the auriculotemporal nerve.

2.2.2 Masseter

The masseter locates superficial to the ramus of mandible, originates from the anterior 2/3 of the lower border and the deep surface of the zygomatic arch. Its muscular fibers are mainly inserted into the masseteric tuberosity. The superficial portion of the parotid gland covers the posterosuperior part of the muscle. The parotid duct, the transverse facial vessels, as well as the buccal and mandibular branches of facial nerve pass across the surface of the masseter.

Section 2

Dissection and observation

Ⅰ. Position and incisions

Place the cadaver in the supine position and put a block under the neck to raise the head for convenience of operation.

● Make a median sagittal incision through the skin of the scalp from the external occipital protuberance to the root of the nose. Make a circular incision around the margins of nostrils and lips, finally extends incision to the mental protuberance of the mandible.

● Make a coronal incision from the middle of the sagittal incision on vertex to the top of the root of auricle.

● Make a transverse skin incision from the root of nose, around the superior, inforior free margins of the eyelids to the front of earlobe.

● Make another transverse incision from the chin to the mastoid process along the lower border and the angle of mandible.

Ⅱ. Procedures

1 The layers of the scalp in the fronto-parieto-occipital region

Strip the skin downward from the central of the cranial vault. The fibrous bands connecting the skin and the epicranial aponeurosis result in difficulty of reflexion.

1. 1 Dissect structures in the superficial fascia

Review the structures such as the supratrochlear nerve and vessels, the supraorbital vessels and nerve.

Trace the temporal branch of the facial nerve upward and expose the anterior part of the temporal fascia.

Trace the superficial temporal vessels and the auriculotemporal nerve.

Find the great auricular nerve, the lesser occipital nerve, the posterior auricular vessels and nerve which behind the root of auricule.

Cut the superficial fascia along the same incisures as skin and turn them laterally and downward, avoid injuring the vessels and nerve.

1.2　Observe the epicranial aponeurosis

The epicranial aponeurosis connects with the frontal belly anteriorly and the occipital belly posteriorly.

1.3　Dissect the subaponeurotic loose connective tissue

Cut the epicranial aponeurosis along the same incisures and insert the handle of scalpel into the subaponeurotic loose connective tissue to separate the epicranial aponeurosis from the pericranium.

1.4　Dissect and observe the pericranium

Cut the pericranium along the same incisures with the apex of the scalpel and separate it from the cranium carefully. It connects with the surface of the cranium loosely whereas it is fixed to the sutures tightly.

2　The temporal region

2.1　Observe and dissect the temporal fascia

Cut the temporal fascia vertically inferior to the midpoint of the zygomatic arch. Observe the two layers of its inferior part. The superficial layer connects to the superior margin of the zygomatic arch while the deep layer connects with the fascia beneath the masseter. There are some adipose tissue and the middle temporal vessels between two layers of the temporal fascia. Cut the superficial layer along the superior margin of the zygomatic arch and explore the extension of the deep layer.

2.2　Observe the temporalis

Check the shape, origin and insertion of the temporalis after the dissection of the temporal fascia.

3　Superficial layer of the face

Turn the skin laterally with scalpel from the anterior median line, identify the major muscles of expression.

The circle muscles around eyes and mouth are orbicularis oculi and orbicularis oris, respectively. In addition, some radial muscles are arranged around the mouth, such as the levator labii superioris, depressor labii inferior is and the buccinators.

3.1　Dissect the parotideomasseteric region

3.1.1　Find the parotid gland and its duct

Palpate the parotid gland below the zygomatic arch and at the posterior border of the masseter. The connective tissue covering the gland is parotideomasseteric fascia or the outer layer sheath of parotid gland. Carefully remove the fascia to expose the gland, avoid damaging the great auricular nerve (one cutaneous branch of the cervical plexus ascending to the earlobe almost vertically) and the superficial lymph nodes of the parotid gland (not demanding). Trace the duct from the anterior border of the gland and 1 cm below the zygomatic arch, then follow it to the anterior border of the masseter where it passes through the masseter at a right angle to the oral cavity. Occasionally, there is an accessary parotid gland adjacent to the duct.

3.1.2　Dissect the nerves and vessels passing through the border of the gland

Find the superficial temporal artery, two terminal branches (parietal branch and frontal branch) of the artery and vein. In front of vessels, trace the temporal branch of the facial nerve which emerges at the anterior superior border. The auriculotemporal nerve is posterior to the vessels.

Find out the thin transverse facial artery and the zygomatic branch of the facial nerve between the zygomatic arch and the duct of the parotid gland.

Trace the buccal branch of the facial nerve underneath the duct and at the anterior border of the parotid gland.

At the anterior inferior border of the gland, trace the marginal mandibular branch of the facial nerve which runs along the inferior border of the mandibular body and spans the facial vessels superiorly.

Trace the cervical branch of the facial nerve at the inferior border of the parotid gland.

3.1.3　Dissect and observe the facial nerve, the external carotid artery and the retromandibular vein

Follow the branches of the facial nerve back through the gland to the trunk of nerve and trace them to the stylomastoid foramen. If possible, find out the posterior auricular branch and the branch to stylohyoid which give off deeply to the gland. Disclose the retromandibular vein and the external carotid artery by removing more of the gland. Pay attention to the structures which surround and pass through the gland when you're moving the gland.

3.2　Dissect the facial vessels

Find the facial artery and the facial vein which lies posterior to the artery, at the junction of the lower border of the mandible and the anterior border of masseter. In the course over the face, it passes about a finger's breadth lateral to the angle of mouth and gives off branches to the lips and the nose. The facial vein begins at the medial angle of the eye and runs downward and backward through the face, posterior to the facial artery. Note that the facial vein receives one tributary (the deep facial vein communicating with the pterygoid venous plexus) at the surface of buccinators.

3.3　Dissect the cutaneous branches of the trigeminal nerve and its accompanying vessels

Find the supraorbital vessels and nerve superior to the medial part of the supraorbital margin and trace the nerve downward to the supraorbital foramen, trace the vessels upward to the cranial vault. Look for the supratrochlear nerve medial to the supraorbital vessels and nerve.

Turn the inferior and medial part of the orbicularis oculi and levator labii superioris to expose the infraorbital vessels and nerve which appearing at the infraorbital foramen.

Strip the depressor anguli oris downward at the angle of the mouth, find the mental vessels and nerve appearing at the mental foramen.

Section 3

Clinical application

I. Parotiditis

The infection and pus in parotid spread medially to the parapharyngeal space because the superficial sheath of parotid is thick and strong whereas the deep sheath of it is thin and incomplete.

II. Facial nerve

There are the facial nerve, the retromandibular vein and the external carotid artery in the parotid gland. The facial nerve and all its branches lie in one plane which are just between the superficial part and the deep part of the parotid gland. In the surgical treatment of parotid tumors, it is important to protect aforementioned nerve and vessels.

III. Pterion

The fracture is easily happened on the pterion region because the bony structure of this region is very thin. Furthermore, the large anterior branch of the middle meningeal artery just crosses the pterion. So this artery is tend to be torn by the fracture in the temporal region of the skull and the extradural hematoma may occur.

IV. Basal cell epithelioma

It generally appears on the face, where sweat glands, oil glands, and hair follicles are abundant. It often occur in fair-skinned males over 40. However, it may extend to surrounding normal skin tissue and cause infection and hemorrhage.

Section 4

Ask yourself

1. How to identify the subcutaneous hematoma, subgaleal hematoma and subperioste-al hematoma?

2. Why the subaponeurotic space is called "the risk area"?

3. Why it is more difficult to stanch bleeding for open wounds and injuries of scalp?

4. Where is the dangerous triangle of face? What is its clinical significance?

5. Which vessels and nerves are liable to be influenced when the parotitis or parotid tumor occurred?

6. Please describe the characteristic and clinical significance of the sheath of parotid gland.

Chapter 4
The neck

Section 1

Review

Hyoid bone It lies inferior to the mental protuberance. Its greater horn is the landmark to look for the lingual artery and can be felt on both sides of hyoid bone.

Thyroid cartilage It lies inferior to the hyoid bone. The upper edge is at the level of the 4th cervical vertebra where the common carotid artery divides into the external and internal carotid arteries. The cartilage projects forward as a laryngeal prominence.

Cricoid cartilage It lies inferior to the thyroid cartilage and at the level of the 6th cervical vertebra. The lower border marks the ends of pharynx and larynx, hence the commencements of the esophagus and trachea. It can be used as a sign of thyroid palpation and tracheal ring count.

Sternocleidomastoid It is an important symbol of the neck divisions. The area between the two commencements which called lesser supraclavicular fossa lies above the sternoclavicular joint. The middle of the posterior margin of the muscle is the convergence point of the cutaneous branches of cervical plexus, so here is the place of cervical plexus block anesthesia.

Greater supraclavicular fossa Also known as the supraclavicular triangle, it lies superior to the middle third of the clavicle. The subclavian artery, the brachial plexus and the 1st rib can be felt on the floor of this fossa.

Suprasternal fossa It lies superior to the jugular notch and can be used as the site of tracheal palpation.

Ⅱ. Boundaries and divisions

The neck is bounded superiorly by an imaginary line linking with the lower border of mandible, the angle of mandible, the mastoid process, the superior nuchal line and the external occipital protuberance; inferiorly by the upper border of sternum, the clavicle and a line extending from the acromion to the spine of the 7th cervical vertebra.

The neck can be divided into two parts by the anterior margin of the trapezius. The posterior portion is called the nape, and the anterior portion is called the proper neck. The proper neck is subdivided by the sternocleidomastoid into three regions: the anterior region, the lateral region and the sternocleidomastoid region.

The anterior region of the neck can be subdivided by the hyoid bone into suprahyoid and infrahyoid regions. The suprahyoid region consists of the submental triangle and the submandibular triangle. The infrahyoid region is composed of the carotid triangle and the muscular triangle.

The lateral region of the neck can be subdivided into an upper larger occipital triangle and a lower smaller greater supraclavicular fossa by the inferior belly of the omohyoid.

Ⅲ. Main contents

1　Skin

It is thin, soft and movable.

2　Superficial fascia

The superficial fascia is loose. It contains fat, platysma, superficial veins, nerves and lymph nodes.

2.1　Platysma

The platysma is the expression muscle in the neck which arises from the fasciae of the pectoralis major and deltoid. The platysma crosses the clavicle and inserts into the mandible and subcutaneous tissues of the lower face.

2.2　Superficial veins

The anterior jugular vein lies laterally to the midline of the neck. It runs inferiorly to the suprasternal space where it pierces the deep cervical fascia and ends in the external jugular vein.

The external jugular vein is formed by the union of the posterior branch of the retromandibular vein with the posterior auricular vein. The vein crosses the fascia on the sternocleidomastoid, runs downward to the root of the neck where it ends in the subclavian vein at the posterior border of the sternocleidomastoid.

2.3　Superficial nerves

The cervical branch of the facial nerve pierces the lower margin of the parotid gland. It runs downward deeply to the platysma and supplies this muscle.

The cutaneous branches of the cervical plexus emerge out near the middle of the posterior border of the sternocleidomastoid and distribute fan-shaped to most skin of the anterior part of neck. These branches are the lesser occipital nerve, the greater auricular nerve, the transverse nerve of neck, and the supraclavicular nerve.

3 Cervical fascia and fascial spaces

3.1 Cervical fascia

The cervical fascia which lies deep to the superficial fascia and platysma is comparatively dense. It can be divided into three layers and forms some fascial spaces.

● Superficial layer of the cervical fascia   It is also called the enveloping fascia because it ensheathes the neck like a tube. It is divided into two layers to enclose the sternocleidomastoid, trapezius, the submandibular and parotid glands.

● Middle layer of the cervical fascia   It is also called the pretracheal layer or the visceral fascia. It encloses the thyroid gland, the trachea, the esophagus and other viscera. The part in front of the trachea is called the pretracheal fascia which forms the thyroid sheath. The part posterior to the esophagus extends upward to cover the posterior wall of the pharynx and the surface of the buccinators (this is the buccopharyngeal fascia).

● Deep layer of the cervical fascia   It is also called the prevertebral fascia. It covers the prevertebral muscles, extends from the base of the skull to the 3rd thoracic vertebra, where it fuses with the anterior longitudinal ligament. This layer of cervical fascia also extends downward and laterally from the scalene fissure as the axillary sheath which surrounds the axillary vessels and brachial plexus.

● Carotid sheath   The middle layer of the cervical fascia extends laterally and forms the carotid sheath which encloses the common and internal carotid arteries, the internal jugular vein and the vagus nerve. It extends from the base of the skull to the root of the neck, and connects with the enveloping fascia and prevertebral fascia by loose connective tissue.

3.2 Fascial spaces

● Suprasternal space   Above the upper border of the manubrium sterni, the superficial layer of cervical fascia divides into two layers and attaches to its anterior and posterior margins to form the suprasternal space. The anterior jugular vein, jugular venous arch, sternal head of sternocleidomastoid, lymph nodes and adipose tissue are in it.

● Supraclavicular space   Above the clavicle, the superficial layer of cervical fascia divides into two layers to form the supraclavicular space. It communicates with the suprasternal space behind the sternocleidomastoid and contains external jugular vein and anterior jugular vein.

● Pretracheal space   It lies between pretracheal fascia and trachea. It contains the pretracheal lymph nodes, inferior thyroid vein, unpaired thyroid venous plexus, lowest thyroid artery, brachiocephalic trunk and left brachiocephalic vein.

● Retropharyngeal space   It lies between buccopharyngeal fascia and prevertebral fascia. It contains loose connective tissue. This space extends above to the base of the skull, below to the posterior mediastinum.

● Prevertebral space   It lies between prevertebral fascia and cervical vertebral column.

● Submandibular space   In the submandibular triangle, the superficial layer of cervical fascia divides into two layers to form the submandibular space. It contains the submandibular gland, submandibular lymph nodes, facial artery and facial vein.

4 Submandibular triangle

4.1 Boundaries

It is enclosed by the lower border of the mandible, the anterior and posterior bellies of digastric.

4.2 Contents

4.2.1 Submandibular gland

It is enclosed by enveloping fascia and separated by mylohyoid into a greater superficial part and a smaller deep part. The submandibular duct arises from the deep part and runs forward between mylohyoid and hyoglossus.

4.2.2 Blood supply

● Facial vein   It begins as the angular vein and runs downward and backward through the face. After turning round the lower border of the mandible at the anterior border of the masseter, it appears in the submandibular triangle and runs across the submandibular gland where it joined by the anterior branch of the retromandibular vein and drains into the internal jugular vein.

● Facial artery   It runs upward and forward in deep groove of the submandibular gland, and then hooks around the lower border of the mandible at the anterior border of the masseter to enter the face.

● Lingual artery and vein   They run forward deep to the hyoglossus. At the anterior border of the hyoglossus, it becomes the deep artery and vein of the tongue.

4.2.3 Nerves

● Lingual nerve   It runs forward between the submandibular gland and the hyoglossus.

● Hypoglossal nerve   It runs on the surface of hyoglossus, below the submandibular gland and its duct.

4.2.4 Lymph nodes

There are 4~6 submandibular lymph nodes between the gland and the lower border of the mandible.

5 Muscular triangle

5.1 Boundaries

It is enclosed by the median line of the neck, the superior belly of the omohyoid and the anterior border of the sternocleidomastoid.

5.2 Contents

The contents of this triangle are the infrahyoid muscles, the thyroid gland, the parathyroid gland, the cervical parts of trachea and esophagus etc.

Enclosed in a sheath formed by the pretracheal fascia(the thyroid sheath, false capsule)and its own fibrous capsule(the true capsule), the thyroid gland consists of right and left lobes united by a narrow isthmus that extends across the 2nd~4th rings of trachea. Its lateral lobes overlap the sides of the larynx and trachea and extend from middle of thyroid cartilage to the 5th or 6th tracheal ring.

Anterior of the thyroid gland(from superficial to deep) are the skin, the superficial fascia, the enveloping fascia, the infrahyoid muscles and the pretracheal fascia. The posteromedial aspect of each lobe are the larynx and trachea, the pharynx and esophagus, and the recurrent laryngeal nerve. Lateral to each lobes are the carotid sheath and the sympathetic trunk.

The blood vessels and nerves of the thyroid gland are as follows:

● Superior thyroid artery and superior laryngeal nerve   The superior thyroid artery arises from the external carotid artery. Firstly, it accompanies the superior laryngeal nerve and its external laryngeal nerve, and then leaves the nerve about 1 cm above the superior pole of the gland. It also gives off the superior laryngeal artery which pierces the thyrohyoid membrane in accompany with the internal laryngeal nerve and arrives in the larynx.

● Inferior thyroid artery and recurrent laryngeal nerve   The inferior thyroid artery arises from the thyrocervical trunk of the subclavian artery. It ascends to the level of the cricoid cartilage and then turns medially behind the carotid sheath to the middle of the posterior border of the thyroid gland. The recurrent laryngeal nerve ascends in the groove between the trachea and the esophagus. Near the lower pole of the gland, it may cross in front of or behind the inferior thyroid artery.

● Lowest thyroid artery   It is occasional (6%～13%) unpaired artery arising from the aortic arch or the brachiocephalic trunk. It ascends in front of the trachea to reach the isthmus of the gland.

● Venous drainage   The superior thyroid vein arises from the upper pole of the lateral lobe and runs upward with the superior thyroid artery to drain into the internal jugular vein. The middle thyroid vein arises near the lateral border of the gland and passes across the common carotid artery to enter the internal jugular vein. The inferior thyroid vein arises from the network on the isthmus and opens into the brachiocephalic vein in front of the trachea.

6 Carotid triangle

6.1 Boundaries

It is enclosed by the superior belly of omohyoid, anterior border of the sternocleidomastoid and posterior belly of digastric.

6.2 Contents

6.2.1 Internal jugular vein

It lies deeply to the anterior border of the sternocleidomastoid and receives the blood from the superior and middle thyroid veins, the facial vein and the lingual vein.

6.2.2 Common carotid artery

It lies on the medial side of the internal jugular vein. At the level of the upper border of the thyroid cartilage, the common carotid artery divides into the external and internal carotid arteries. The carotid body (chemical receptor) is on the internal surface of the carotid bifurcation, and the carotid sinus (pressure receptor) lies on the upper end of the common carotid artery and the root of the internal carotid artery. The internal carotid artery has no branch in neck. The branches of the external carotid artery are the superior thyroid, lingual, facial, occipital and posterior auricular arteries.

6.2.3 Nerves

● Hypoglossal nerve It crosses the internal and external carotid arteries and enters the submandibular triangle. Its descending branch (superior root of the ansa cervicalis) joins the anterior branches of the cervical nerves (inferior root of the ansa cervicalis) to form the ansa cervicalis which gives off the branches to innervate the infrahyoid muscles.

● Vagus nerve It lies in the posterior part of the carotid sheath between the internal jugular vein and the common carotid artery. The branches of vagus nerve in the carotid triangle are the superior laryngeal nerve and the cardiac branch. The superior laryngeal nerve divides into internal and external laryngeal nerves which accompany with the superior laryngeal and the superior thyroid arteries to the mucous membrane above the vocal folds and the cricothyroid of the larynx. The cardiac branch goes downward into the thorax to take part in the cardiac plexus.

7 Sternocleidomastoid region

7.1 Boundaries

It is the area occupied and covered by the sternocleidomastoid.

7.2　Contents

7.2.1　Carotid sheath

It begins from the base of the skull and continues with the mediastinum at the root of neck. In the sheath, there are the internal and common carotid arteries on the medial side, the internal jugular vein on the lateral side, and the vagus nerve behind them. Anterior to the sheath, there are the sternohyoid, sternothyroid, omohyoid and the sternocleidomastoid. The ansa cervicalis lies on the surface or in the sheath. Posteriorly, the prevertebral muscles and the sympathetic trunk lie beneath the prevertebral fascia. Medially, there are the larynx, trachea, pharynx, esophagus, recurrent laryngeal nerve, lateral lobe of thyroid gland etc.

7.2.2　Ansa cervicalis

It is formed by the superior root (arises from the hypoglossal nerve) and the inferior root (arises from the anterior branches of the cervical nerves) at the level of the lower border of the larynx. It sends branches to innervate the infrahyoid muscles.

7.2.3　Cervical plexus

It is formed by the anterior branches of the upper four cervical nerves and lies under the upper half of the sternocleidomastoid. The branches of the cervical plexus are the cutaneous branches, muscular branches and the phrenic nerve.

7.2.4　Cervical portion of the sympathetic trunk

The sympathetic trunk lies on both sides of the cervical vertebral column and is covered by the prevertebral fascia. It is formed by the paravertebral ganglia (superior, middle, inferior ganglia) and the interganglionic fibers. Each ganglion gives off a cardiac branch to join the deep cardiac plexus.

8　Greater supraclavicular fossa

8.1　Boundaries

The greater supraclavicular fossa is bounded anteriorly by the posterior border of the sternocleidomastoid, posteriorly by the inferior belly of the omohyoid, and inferiorly by the middle third of the clavicle.

8.2　Contents

In this fossa, the scalenus anterior is the key mark to identify the relationships of other structures. Anteriorly, there are the internal jugular vein, phrenic nerve, transverse cervical artery, suprascapular artery, subclavian vein and the thoracic duct. Posteriorly, the second part of the subclavian artery and the roots and trunks of the brachial plexus are located in the scalene fissure. Posteromedially, there are the cupula of pleura and the apex of the lung.

8.2.1 Phrenic nerve

It arises from the cervical plexus and descends over the front of the scalenus anterior deep to the prevertebral fascia, then passes onto the cupula of pleura between the subclavian artery and vein to enter the thorax.

8.2.2 Subclavian vein

It continues with the axillary vein and runs medially over the front of the scalenus anterior and the cupula of pleura. At the medial border of the scalenus anterior, it unites the internal jugular vein to form the brachiocephalic vein. The angle of the union is termed the venous angle.

8.2.3 Subclavian artery

It arches laterally across the front of the cupula of pleura and passes in the scalene fissure to the outer border of the 1st rib, where it becomes the axillary artery.

8.2.4 Brachial plexus

It lies behind the cupula of pleura and the subclavian artery and runs laterally in the scalene fissure to enter the axillary fossa. The branches of the supraclavicular part of the brachial plexus are the suprascapular, the dorsal scapular and the long thoracic nerves.

9 Occipital triangle

9.1 Boundaries

It is bounded by the posterior border of the sternocleidomastoid, anterior border of the trapezius, and the inferior belly of the omohyoid.

9.2 Contents

The main contents of this triangle are the spinal accessory nerve, lateral cervical lymph nodes and some cutaneous branches of the cervical plexus.

Section 2

Dissection and observation

Ⅰ. Position and incisions

Place the cadaver in the supine position. Put a block under the shoulders, or let the head hang over the edge of the autopsy table in order to extend the head and neck as much as possible.

Make a median skin incision from the midpoint of base of mandible to the jugular notch of sternum.

From the upper end of the median incision, make a transverse incision along the lower border of the mandible to the mastoid process.

From the lower end of the median incision, make another transverse incision along the upper border of the clavicle to the acromion.

Ⅱ. Procedures

1 Dissect superficial structures of the neck

1.1 Dissect the platysma

Strip the skin flaps laterally to the anterior border of the trapezius. Observe the platysma, cut it from the upper border of the clavicle and turn it upward to the mandible. Look for the cervical branch of the facial nerve which innervates this muscle.

1.2 Dissect the superficial veins

On both sides of the median line in the superficial fascia, identify the anterior jugular veins and trace them downward until they pierce the deep fascia. Then, identify the external jugular vein on the surface of the sternocleidomastoid, trace it to the deep fascia.

1.3 Dissect the cutaneous branches of the cervical plexus

Near the midpoint of the posterior border of the sternocleidomastoid, identify and trace the cutaneous branches of the cervical plexus. The greater auricular nerve runs upward. Trace it to the auricle and parotid region. The transverse nerve of neck crosses the sternocleidomastoid horizontally and runs forward. The lesser occipital nerve runs upward along the posterior border of the sternocleidomastoid to the mastoid process. Look for the supraclavicular nerves descending laterally and trace them downward to the pectoral and shoulder region.

Reserve aforementioned superficial veins and cutaneous nerves, clean the superficial fascia.

2　Dissect and observe the cervical fascia

2.1　Observe the enveloping fascia

It is attached to the upper and lower margins of the neck. It encloses the trapezius, the sternocleidomastoid, the submandibular and parotid glands.

2.2　Dissect the enveloping fascia and jugular arch

Cut the anterior layer of the enveloping fascia above the sternum and expose the suprasternal space. Dissect the jugular venous arch which is formed by right and left anterior jugular veins.

2.3　Dissect the sternocleidomastoid

Remove the enveloping fascia from the surface of the sternocleidomastoid to its posterior border. Secure the external jugular vein and the cutaneous branches of the cervical plexus. Sever the origins of this muscle and pull them upward. Look for the accessory nerve which innervates this muscle.

2.4　Dissect the infrahyoid muscles and ansa cervicalis

Clean the enveloping fascia below the hyoid bone to expose the infrahyoid muscles. Observe the middle layer of the cervical fascia which encloses these muscles. Separate the infrahyoid muscles and look for the nerves innervating them. Trace these nerves to the ansa cervicalis which usually lies in front of the carotid sheath. Push the carotid sheath medially and observe the deep layer of the cervical fascia (prevertebral fascia).

3　Dissect the muscular triangle

Transect the sternohyoid and sternothyroid near their lower ends and turn them upward respectively.

Examine the pretracheal fascia (visceral fascia). It encloses the thyroid gland and forms the false capsule. Observe the shape and location of the lateral lobes, the isthmus and the pyramidal lobe of the thyroid gland.

Look for the superior thyroid artery and vein near the upper pole of the lateral lobe of the gland. Trace them upward to the external carotid artery and internal jugular vein respectively. Look for the branch of superior thyroid artery, the superior laryngeal artery, which accompanies with the internal branch of superior laryngeal nerve to pierce the thyrohyoid memebrane. Look for the external branch of superior laryngeal nerve to the cricothyroid muscle.

In the pretracheal space, identify the lowest thyroid artery and the inferior thyroid vein.

Find the middle thyroid vein on the lateral side of the lower part of the lateral lobe. Trace it to the internal jugular vein. Cut this vein and pull the lateral lobe medially to expose the back of the gland. Find the inferior thyroid artery near the lower pole. Look for the recurrent laryngeal nerve which lies in the groove between the trachea and esophagus. Note the close relationship between the recurrent laryngeal nerve and the inferior thyroid artery.

In front of the thyroid gland, cut through the thyroid sheath(false capsule) strip the flaps to expose the fibrous capsule (true capsule). Identify the suspensory ligament of thyroid which is attached to the cartilage of larynx and the most upper cartilage of the trachea. Find the parathyroid glands along the posterior surface of the lateral lobe of thyroid gland between the capsule and sheath.

4 Dissect the carotid triangle and the sternocleidomastoid region

4. 1 Dissect the carotid sheath

Observe the ansa cervicalis. Identify its superior root (the descending branch of the hypoglossal nerve) and the inferior root (from the anterior branches of the second and third cervical nerves). Cut the sheath longitudinally and identify the relationship among the internal jugular vein, internal carotid artery and the common carotid artery. Examine the carotid sinus and carotid body near the bifurcation of the common carotid artery.

4. 2 Dissect the internal jugular vein and hypoglossal nerve

In the upper part of the carotid triangle, find out the (common) facial vein that ends in the internal jugular vein. Look for the hypoglossal nerve which crosses the internal and external carotid arteries at the lower border of the posterior belly of the digastric. It also can be found by tracing the superior root of the ansa cervicalis. Trace the hypoglossal nerve to submandibular triangle.

4. 3 Dissect the branches of the external carotid artery

Trace the superior thyroid artery to the external carotid artery. On top of this artery, search the lingual and facial arteries and trace them upward deep to the posterior belly of the digastric.

4. 4 Dissect the vagus nerve

Isolate the internal jugular vein from the carotid arteries and find the vagus nerve in the posterior part of the sheath. Trace the internal and external branches of superior laryngeal nerve upward to the superior laryngeal nerve, and then to the vagus nerve.

4. 5 Dissect the phrenic nerve

Remove the carotid sheath. Detach the prevertebral fascia from the anterior surface of the scalenus anterior and expose the phrenic nerve. Trace the nerve upward and downward.

4. 6 Dissect the sympathetic trunk

Pull the internal jugular vein, carotid arteries and the vagus nerve laterally. Along the sides of vertebral bodies and deep to the prevertebral fascia, expose the sympathetic trunk and trace it upward and downward. Pay attention to the cervical ganglia and the cardiac branch on it.

5 Dissect the submental triangle

Observe the boundaries of this triangle. In the enveloping fascia, look for the submental lymph nodes (one or two) and remove them. Clean the mylohyoid and the anterior belly of digastric.

6 Dissect the submandibular triangle

Clear the enveloping fascia to expose the submandibular gland. At the anteroinferior angle of the masseter, identify the facial artery and facial vein. Follow the facial vein downward and backward across the gland and the posterior belly of digastric. Trace the facial artery downward and backward deep to the gland. Raise the gland upward to observe the intermediate tendon of the digastric and the stylohyoid.

Cut the origin of the anterior belly of digastric and turn it downward. Clean the mylohyoid and cut it along the median line. On the surface of the hyoglossus, identify the hypoglossal nerve and trace it backward and upward.

Between the hypoglossal nerve and the greater horn of the hyoid, search the lingual artery and vein.

7 Dissect the lateral region

7. 1 Examine the boundaries of the lateral region of the neck

Replace the sternocleidomastoid to define the boundaries of the lateral region of the neck (posterior triangle). Look for the inferior belly of the omohyoid which divides this region into two parts: the occipital triangle and the greater supraclavicular fossa.

7. 2 Dissect the accessory nerve

Under the enveloping fascia, search the accessory nerve at the junction of the upper and middle thirds of the posterior border of sternocleidomastoid. It runs obliquely downward to end in the trapezius at the junction of the middle and lower thirds of its anterior border. Trace the accessory nerve and look for its muscular branches which innervate the trapezius and sternocleidomastoid.

7.3 Dissect the brachial plexus

Clean the scalenus anterior and medius. Identify the scalene fissure between these two muscles. Then, look for the roots, trunks, divisions of the brachial plexus and trace them to the axillary fossa. Look for the suprascapular nerve arising from the upper trunk or its posterior division. Search the dorsal scapular nerve which arises from the root of C5. Look for the long thoracic nerve between the plexus and the scalenus medius. It arises from the root of C5 – C7 and enters the axilla behind the first part of the axillary artery.

7.4 Dissect the muscles

Clean the muscles of the lateral region. Observe the scalenus medius, scalenus posterior and levator scapulae.

8 Dissect the root of the neck

8.1 Remove the clavicle

Separate the sternoclavicular joint with knife and cut the clavicle between its middle and lateral thirds with saw. Detach the subclavius from the clavicle carefully and remove the isolated part of the clavicle.

8.2 Dissect the venous angle and the lymphatic duct

Clean the internal jugular vein, subclavian vein and the brachiocephalic vein. At the junction of the subclavian and internal jugular veins (venous angle), search and trace the thoracic duct (left side) and the right lymphatic duct (right side).

8.3 Dissect the vagus nerve

Clean the common carotid artery and the subclavian artery. Trace the vagus nerve downward between the common carotid artery and the internal jugular vein to the thorax. Look for and define the right recurrent laryngeal nerve which loops below and behind the subclavian artery, ascends obliquely to the posteriolateral aspect of the trachea and passes upward toward the larynx.

8.4 Dissect the subclavian artery

On the medial side of the scalenus anterior, clean the first part of the subclavian artery and its branches, the vertebral artery, thyrocervical trunk and the internal thoracic artery. Examine the relations of the subclavian artery. Anteriorly, the internal jugular vein, vertebral vein, vagus nerve and phrenic nerve run across it. The brachial plexus is superior and posterior to the artery. Identify the branches of the thyrocervical trunk. They are the inferior thyroid, the suprascapular and the transverse cervical arteries.

Section 3

Clinical application

Incision on mandibular brunch of the facial nerve

A transverse incision just below the mandible can occasionally induce injury to the marginal mandibular branch of the facial nerve. It will result in a disfiguring ipsilateral mouth droop.

II. Drainage of pus

The collections of pus dorsal to the prevertebral fascia may form a mid-line swelling behind the posterior wall of the pharynx. The abscess may then track laterally deep to the carotid sheath, to a point behind the sternocleidomastoid. Rarely, pus may travel along the axillary sheath into the arm, or along the prevertebral space into the mediastinum.

Ligature of blood vessels in thyroidectomy

● Incision   A transverse "collar" incision is carried out along the skin crease about 2 finger's breadth above the jugular notch. For a better exposure of the thyroid gland, the sternohyoid and sternothyroid with their enveloping fascia should be transected at their upper extremities because the nerves enter the inferior part of the muscles.

● Ligature of the superior thyroid artery   The external laryngeal nerve is not so closely related to the superior thyroid artery as it is at its origin. Therefore, this artery should be ligated near the upper pole of the thyroid gland.

● Ligature of the inferior thyroid artery   Near the lower third of the lateral lobe of the gland, the right recurrent laryngeal nerve is closely related to the inferior thyroid artery. It may cross anterior or posterior to the artery. Therefore, the inferior thyroid artery should be ligated some distance lateral to the thyroid gland. Left recurrent laryngeal nerve is deeper in the tracheoesophageal groove and always located behind the inferior thyroid artery, so that the danger of injuring the left nerve is not so great as the right one.

IV. Tracheotomy incision

In front of the trachea, there are the isthmus of thyroid, the inferior thyroid veins, and the lowest thyroid artery. The common carotid artery is more close to the trachea inferiorly. In children, some other structures, such as the thymus, left brachiocephalic vein, the brachiocephalic trunk, even the aortic arch may be above the jugular notch of sternum. Therefore, more attention should be paid to the tracheotomy in children. The principles are as follows.

● The neck should be fully extended and the head is held exactly in the median line.

● In order to protect the structures above the jugular notch of sternum, the incision of the trachea should be made above the 5th tracheal ring. Usually, it is made through the 2nd and 3rd tracheal ring.

● The trachea of infants is softer than that of the adult. Do not pierce its posterior wall and damage the underlying esophagus.

Section 4

Ask yourself

1. Which structures would be gone through in thyroid surgery? Which structures should be ligated? Which vulnerable organs should be protected?

2. Which structures are easily compressed in goiter?

3. Which structures need to be carefully separated in tracheotomy? What should be pay attention to?

4. Which nervous plexus should be blocked when operation on the anterolateral part of the neck?

5. How to distinguish the internal carotid from external carotid arteries during the surgery?

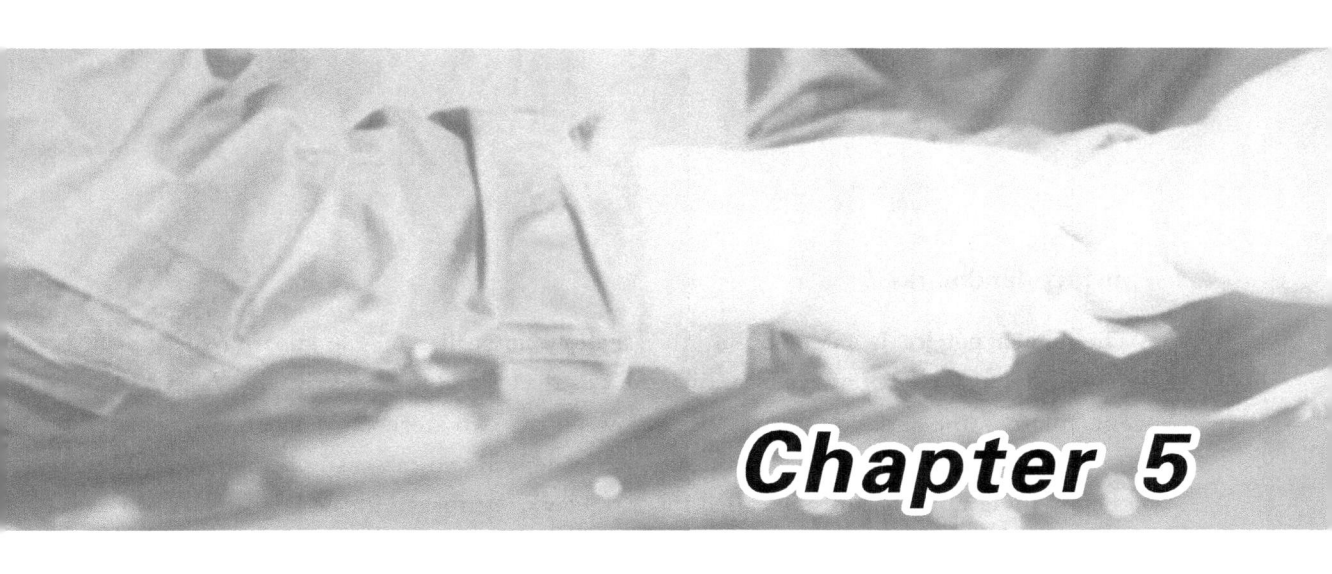

Chapter 5

The thorax

Section 1

Review

Ⅰ. Surface anatomy

1 Surface landmarks

The **jugular notch**　In male adults, this shallow notch lies on the superior margin of the manubrium at the level of the inferior border of the second thoracic vertebra body. Just above it, there is the superior sternal fossa between the two sternocleidomastoid muscles.

The **clavicle**　It is subcutaneous throughout its length and can easily be palpated. The fossa below its lateral one third is called the infraclavicular fossa. In the lateral part of the fossa, the coracoid process can be palpated 1 finger below the clavicle.

The **sternal angle**　(also known as the angle of Louis or manubriosternal junction) It is a palpated transverse ridge on the anterior surface of sternum at the junction of the manubrium with the body of the sternum. It is slightly convex forward and easily palpated even in obesity group. It marks the approximate level of the second pair of costal cartilages, which attach to the 2nd ribs and makes it possible to identify and locate the other ribs below the second.

The **xiphoid process**　It is the inferior part of the of the sternum. The xiphosternal synchondrosis where the xiphoid process fused with the sternal body connects the 7th costal cartilage on both sides.

The **costal margin (costal arch)**　It is formed by the 7th to the 10th costal cartilages. The costal margin is usually used as a surface marker for the liver, gallbladder and spleen in clinical palpation.

The **infrasternal angle**　It is composed of bilateral costal arch and xiphosternal synchondrosis. It is about 70~110 degree angel opening downward. There is a xiphocostal angle formed by the xiphoid process and the costal arch on each side. The left xiphocostal angle is the location where pericardiocentesis is carried out usually.

The **nipple**　In the male, the nipple usually lies in the 4th intercostal space about 10 cm from the midline. In the female, its position is not constant due to the different shapes of breasts.

The **inferior angle of scapula**　It lies on the opposite side of 7th rib or 7th intercostal space, and can be used for counting the ribs and intercostal spaces.

2　Orientational lines on the thoracic wall

The **anterior median line**　It is the anterior median line over the sternum.

The **sternal line**　It is the vertical line just lateral to the widest part of the sternum.

The **midclavicular line**　It runs vertically through the midpoint of the clavicle.

The **parasternal line**　It is the vertical line through the midway between the sternal line and the midclavicular line.

The **anterior axillary line**　It is the vertical extension line of the anterior axillary fold.

The **posterior axillary line**　It is the vertical extension line of the posterior axillary fold.

The **midaxillary line**　It is the vertical line through the midway between the anterior and posterior axillary folds.

The **scapular line**　It is the vertical line through the inferior angle of the scapula.

The **posterior median line**　It is the vertical through the tips of the spinous processes of the vertebrae.

Ⅱ. Boundaries and divisions

1　Boundaries

Continued with the neck, the thorax is the superior part of the trunk, which is separated from the abdomen by the diaphragm. Its upper boundary (the superior aperture or inlet of the thorax) is formed by a line drawing from the jugular notch, along the superior margins of the clavicles to the acromia on both sides, and then to the spinous processes of the 7th cervical vertebra posteriorly. The lower boundary (the inferior aperture or outlet of the thorax) is formed by a line connecting the xiphoid process, the costal margin and the free borders of 11th and 12th ribs on both sides and the spinous process of the 12th thoracic vertebra posteriorly. The lateral boundaries of the thorax are the anterior and posterior margins of the deltoid which separates the thorax and the upper limbs.

2　Divisions

The thorax consists of the thoracic wall, the thoracic cavity and organs inside the thoracic cavity.

2. 1　Thoracic wall

The thoracic wall is composed of the thoracic cage and soft tissue such as skin, fasciae, muscles, blood vessels and nerves. Each side of thoracic wall can be divided into three regions—the anterior thoracic region is located between the anterior median and the anterior axillary lines, the lateral thoracic region between the anterior and posterior axillary lines and the thoracodorsal region between the posterior axillary and the posterior median lines.

2.2 Thoracic cavity

It is divided into three parts: the left thoracic cavity, the right thoracic cavity and the mediastinum.

III. Main contents

1 Thoracic wall

1.1 Skin

The skin varies in the texture, which is easy to move except the anterior region of the sternum.

1.2 Superficial fascia

It is composed of adipose tissue and connective tissue, and it contains the superficial blood vessels, lymphatic vessels and the cutaneous nerves.

1.2.1 Superficial blood supply

● Arteries   They are the perforating branches of the internal thoracic artery, the lateral and posterior cutaneous branches of the posterior intercostal arteries.

● Veins   The superficial veins anastomose with each other to form venous network in the superficial fascia and finally merge to form the thoracoepigastric vein which runs downward to connect with the venous network around the umbilicus. Upward, they drain into the axillary vein by way of the lateral thoracic vein.

The perforating branches of the internal thoracic vein and the lateral cutaneous branches of the posterior intercostal veins accompanied the corresponding arteries.

1.2.2 Cutaneous nerves

They are the supraclavicular nerve, anterior and lateral cutaneous branches of the intercostal nerves. The supraclavicular nerve is divided into the medial, middle and lateral branches. The distribution level of the intercostal nerves are listed in the below table.

Table 5 - 1 The distribution level of the intercostal nerve

intercostal nerve	2nd	4nd	6nd	8nd	10nd	12th
distribution level	sternal angle	nipple	xiphosternal synchondrosis	costal margin	umbilicus	anterior superior iliac spine

1.2.3　The breast (mamma)

▶ Position

The pair of female breasts are located in superficial fascia between the 2th and 6th ribs on both sides. The medial boundary of each breast is sternal line, and the lateral boundary goes closely to the midaxillary line.

▶ Formation

The breast is composed of the skin, mammary gland, adipose tissue and fibrous connective tissue. Each breast consists of 15-20 lobes of mammary gland, which are composed of the lobules. The mammary glands are separated by the fibrous septa formed by the fibrous tissue. The septa are well developed and extend from the skin, superficial to the deep fascia. The terminal linked with the deep fascia is called the suspensory ligament of breast (Cooper's ligament).

▶ Blood supply

● Arteries　The medial part of the breast is supplied by the perforating branches of the internal thoracic artery passing through the 3rd to 6th intercostal spaces. The lateral part is supplied by the following arteries: the lateral cutaneous branches of the 3rd to 7th posterior intercostal arteries, the branches of the thoracoacromial artery and the lateral thoracic artery.

● Veins　The majority of the superficial veins of the breast drain into the internal thoracic vein and a few into the anterior jugular vein. The deep veins its corresponding drain into the internal thoracic vein, axillary vein, and posterior intercostal veins, respectively.

▶ Lymphatic drainage

The superficial lymphatic plexus is distributed in the skin and the subcutaneous tissue. These superficial lymphatic vessels have no valves and drain into the deep lymphatic vessels or into the pectoral lymph nodes.

The deep lymphatic vessels distribute in the intervals of the lobules and in the wall of the lactiferous ducts. There are four pathways for deep lymphatic drainage: the lymphatic vessels of the lateral and upper parts drain into the anterior group of axillary lymph nodes (pectoral lymph nodes) and their efferent vessels drain into the apical lymph nodes. The lymphatic vessels of the medial part piercing the 1st to 5th intercostal space near the sternum drain into the parasternal lymph nodes along the internal thoracic vessels and their efferent vessels drain into the anterior mediastinal lymph nodes or supraclavicular lymph nodes. These lymphatic vessels may anastomose with the contralateral lymphatic vessels. The lymphatic vessels of the inferomedial part anastomose with the vessels of the anterior abdominal wall and with the subdiaphragmatic and hepatic lymphatic vessels. The deep lymphatic vessels of the breast pierce the pectoralis major and minor directly and drain into the apical lymph nodes. There are lymph nodes located between the pectoralis major and minor, and deep to the pectoralis minor.

1.3 Deep fascia

The deep fascia in the anterior and lateral regions of the thoracic wall may be divided into the superficial and deep layers. The deep layer encloses the subclavius and forms the clavipectoral fascia between the subclavius, the upper border of the pectoralis minor. Deep to the clavipectoral fascia, the lateral pectoral nerve, thoracoacromial vessels pass through the fascia and ends at pectoralis major. And the cephalic vein and lymphatic vessels pierce the fascia into the axilla.

1.4 Muscles

The muscles of the anterior thoracic wall are the pectoralis major, subclavius, pectoralis minor. In the lateral region of the thoracic wall, there are the serratus anterior and the obliquus externus abdominis. In the thoracodorsal region of the thoracic wall, there are the trapezius, rhomboideus and latissimus dorsi. In the inner surface of the lower part of the anterior region of the thoracic wall, there is the transversus thoracis. The rectus abdominis arises from the outer surface of the low part of the anterior region of the thoracic wall. In addition, the intercostal muscles lie in the intercostal space between two adjacent ribs.

1.5 Intercostal spaces

In each thoracic wall, there are 11 intercostal space between 12 ribs.

1.5.1 Intercostal muscles

There are three incomplete layers of muscles in each intercostal space. They are the intercostales externi, the intercostales interni and the intercostales intimi from superficial to deep.

1.5.2 Intercostal nerves and vessels

● Intercostal nerves   The ventral rami of the 1st to 11th thoracic spinal nerves are called the intercostal nerves and the ventral ramus of the 12th thoracic spinal nerve is called the subcostal nerve.

● Intercostal vessels   They are the 11 pairs of posterior intercostal arteries and one pair of subclavian arteries.

The posterior intercostal veins accompany the posterior intercostal arteries. The upper two or three posterior intercostal veins unite into the superior intercostal vein which enters the brachiocephalic vein. The other posterior intercostal veins enter the azygos, hemiazygos or accessory hemiazygos veins.

In the costal groove of the rib, the arrangement from up downward is the vein, artery and nerve.

1.5.3 Internal thoracic vessels

The internal thoracic artery arises at the root of the neck from the first part of the subclavian artery. It ends by dividing into the superior epigastric and musculophrenic arteries at the level of 6th intercostal space. Its branches are the:

- Pericardiacophrenic artery
- Anterior intercostal branches
- Perforating branches
- Superior epigastric artery
- Musculophrenic artery

Furthermore, the internal thoracic artery also has many branches to the sternum and thymus.

The internal thoracic veins accompany the internal thoracic arteries and drain the territory supplied by the internal thoracic arteries. On the right side, the internal thoracic vein enters the junction of the brachiocephalic vein and superior vena cava. And on the left side, it drains into the brachiocephalic vein.

1.6　Endothoracic fascia

It is a thin but dense connective tissue membrane which varies in different regions. It line inner surface of the thoracic wall and upper surface of the diaphragm.

Following structures must be passed through for operation on pleural cavity: the skin, superficial fascia, deep fascia and superficial muscles of the thoracic wall, rib and intercostal muscles, endothoracic fascia and parietal pleura.

2　Diaphragm

2.1　Position and divisions

The diaphragm is dome-shaped musculotendinous septum separating the thoracic cavity from the abdominal cavity. It forms the floor of the thorax and the roof of the abdomen.

The diaphragm consists of a central aponeurotic portion called the central tendon and a peripheral muscular part which fibers are divided into three parts: the sternal part, the costal part, the lumbar part (medial arcuate ligament) and the lateral arcuate ligament). The three parts of the muscular fibers insert into the central tendon.

2.2　Triangles of the diaphragm

Among the three original parts of the diaphragm, there are three triangular spaces without muscular fibers: the anteromedian triangle, the sternocostal triangle and the lumbocostal triangle.

2.3　Openings of the diaphragm

There are three openings in the diaphragm where some blood vessels, lymphatic vessels and nerves pass through.

The aortic hiatus lies at the level of the 12th thoracic vertebrae, slightly to the left of the median plane. The abdominal aorta, the azygos vein and the thoracic duct transmit the hiatus.

The esophageal hiatus is located in the right curs of the diaphragm, 2-3 cm to the left of the median plane, approximately at the level of the 10th thoracic vertebra. The esophagus, esophageal branches of the left gastric vessels and two vagal trunks pass through the hiatus.

The vena caval foramen lies in the central tendon of the diaphragm, at the level of the 8th thoracic vertebra or the intervertebral disc between the 8th and 9th thoracic vertebrae, 2-3 cm to the right of the median plane. The inferior vena cava, the terminal branches of the right phrenic verve and some lymphatic vessels from the liver pass through the foramen.

Besides, the sympathetic trunks pass through the diaphragm posterior to the medial arcuate ligaments, the greater and lesser splanchnic nerves pierce the crura and the hemiazygos vein transmits the left crus.

3 Pleura and pleural cavity

3.1 Pleura

The pleura is an extremly thin serous membrane which has excretive and absorptive function. It envelops the pleural cavity. The pleura consists of the visceral (or pulmonary) and parietal pleurae. The visceral pleura is adherent to the surface of the lung and dips into the pulmonary fissures. The parietal pleura can be subdivided into four parts according to the lining locations: the costal pleura, the diaphragmatic pleura, the cupula (dome) of the pleura (or cervical pleura) and the mediastinal pleura. The visceral and parietal pleurae are continuous with each other around the root of the lung. Below the root of the lung, the mediastinal pleura extends laterally as double layer from the esophagus to the root of the lung, where it is continuous with the visceral pleura. The double layer is called the pulmonary ligament, which fix the lung to the mediastinum.

3.2 Pleural cavity

It is a potential space containing a capillary layer of serous lubricating fluid.

3.3 Pleura recesses

The acute angle, formed by two different parts of parietal pleura, which can not be occupied by expanded lung and are called the pleural recesses. They are the costodiaphragmatic recess, the costomediastinal recess and the phrenicomediastinal recess just on the left side.

3.4 Pleural reflections

The parietal pleura is sharply folded where the costal pleura meets the diaphragmatic pleura, and where the costal pleura meets the mediastinal pleura. The folds are called lines of pleural reflection. The line where the costal meets the diaphragmatic pleurae is called the inferior border of the pleura (costal reflection). The line where the anterior margin of the mediastinal pleura meets the costal pleura is called the anterior border of the pleura (sternal reflection).

Above the sternal angle and below the level of the 4th costal cartilage, the distance between two sternal reflections is larger. These two intervals are called the superior intermediate region (triangle of thymus) and the inferior intermediate region (triangle of pericardium) of the pleura respectively.

4　Lungs

4.1　Position and external features

Separated by mediastinum, the lungs occupy most of the space in the thoracic cavity. The lung, half conical in shape, has an apex, a base, two surfaces and three borders.

4.2　Surface projections

The anterior borders of the lungs are quite alike the sternal reflection of the pleura, except the anterior border of the left lung at the level of the 4th sternocostal joint sharply turns laterally and then descends along the 4th costal cartilage towards the midpoint of the 6th costal cartilage where the anterior border meets the inferior border. The inferior borders of the lungs are slightly higher than the inferior borders of the pleurae (Table 5 – 2). The inferior borders of the lungs vary 2-3 cm upward or downward in inspiration and expiration.

Table 5 – 2　The surface projection of the lungs and pleurae

	Midclavicular line	Midaxillary line	Scapular line	Posterior median line
Inferior order of lungs	6th rib	8th rib	10th rib	The spinous process of the 10th thoracic vertebra.
Inferior order of the pleura	8th rib	10th rib	11th rib	The spinous process of the 12th thoracic vertebra.

4.3　Fissures and lobes

The left lung is divided into two lobes by the oblique fissure. The oblique fissure extends into the lung almost to hilum, and separated the superior and inferior lobes. Besides the oblique fissure, the upper portion of the right lung is divided by a horizontal fissure into superior and middle lobes.

4.4　Bronchopulmonary segments

Each principal bronchus bifurcates secondary(for lobar) bronchi to the lobes of the lung. The lobar bronchus continuously branches tertiary (for segmental) bronchi. Each segmental bronchus with its linked pulmonary tissue is called a bronchopulmonary segment (pulmonary segment). Each pulmonary segment has its own segmental bronchus, artery and vein, it is pyramidal-shaped with its apex towards the hilum of the lung and the base to the surface of the lung.

4.5 Hilum and root

The hilum of the lung may be divided into the primary and secondary pulmonary hila. The primary (first) pulmonary hilum lies near the center of the medial surface of the lung, where the bronchi, pulmonary vessels, bronchial vessels, lymph vessels and nerves enter and leave the lung. The root of the lung is formed by the principal bronchus, the pulmonary veins, the bronchial branches (arteries) and veins, the pulmonary plexuses of nerves and lymphatic vessels. These structures are held together by mediastinal connective tissue and surround by the pleura. The chief structures composing the root of each lung are arranged in a similar manner from anterior to posterior on both sides, they are the pulmonary vein, the pulmonary artery and the bronchus, with the bronchial vessels on its posterior aspect behind. However, their arrangement differs from above downward on the two sides: on the right, their arrangement is superior lobar bronchus, pulmonary artery, middle and inferior lobar bronchus, and pulmonary vein; on the left, they are the pulmonary artery, the bronchus, and pulmonary vein.

4.6 Blood supply, lymphatic drainage and innervation

● Pulmonary artery   The pulmonary trunk derived from the conus arteriosus (infundibulum) of the right ventricle, bifurcates right and left pulmonary arteries under the aortic arch.

● Pulmonary vein   The pulmonary veins drain oxygenated blood from the lung to the left atrium of the heart. They have no valve. Beginning in the pulmonary capillaries, the veins constantly unite into larger and larger veins. Finally the larger veins form the superior and inferior pulmonary veins on each side. They open onto the posterior wall of the left atrium.

● Bronchial arteries   The two left bronchial artery, arise from the front wall of the thoracic aorta. The single or two-branches of the right bronchial artery is generally derived from the right 3rd posterior intercostal artery.

● Bronchial veins   The bronchial veins drain the larger subdivisions of the bronchi and receive twigs from other structures of the posterior mediastinum. The right bronchial vein enters the azygos vein as it arches over the root of the right lung. The left bronchial vein drains into the accessary hemiazygos vein. Inside the lungs, the bronchial veins anastomose with the pulmonary veins.

● Lymphatic drainage   The lymphatic vessels of the lungs are divided into the superficial and deep plexuses.

● Nerve plexuses of the lungs   The nerve plexuses of lungs consist of the anterior pulmonary and posterior pulmonary plexuses, which lie before and behind the root of the lungs respectively.

5   Mediastinum

All the organs and structures between the mediastinal pleura are called the mediastinum. It consists of the pericardium, heart, great vessels, trachea, principal bronchi, esophagus, thymus, thoracic duct, azygos vein, phrenic and vagus nerves, sympathetic trunk and so on.

5.1   Position and boundaries

The superior boundary of the mediastinum is the inlet of the thorax, and the inferior sits on the diaphragm. The sternum and costal cartilages lie in front of the mediastinum, and the thoracic vertebrae lie behind. The lateral boundaries are the mediastinal pleura on both sides. The mediastinum takes up a position of the median portion of the thoracic cavity in childhood, but it slightly bulges to the left side in adults.

5.2   Divisions

In order to facilitate the description of the mediastinum, it is divided by an imaginary horizontal plane from the sternal angel to the lower border of 4th thoracic vertebrae. The portion above this plane is the superior mediastinum. Below this plane, the inferior mediastinum is subdivided into:

● Middle mediastinum   It lies between the coronal plane of the anterior and posterior borders of the pericardium, which consists of the heart in the pericardium with a phrenic nerve on each side and the roots of the great blood vessels.

● Anterior mediastinum   It lies between the anterior border of the pericardium and the sternum.

● Posterior mediastinum   It lies between the posterior border of the pericardium and the thoracic vertebrae.

5.3   The superior mediastinum

The main organs from anterior to posterior are: ① the thymus-vein layer, the thymus or its remnant, right and left brachiocephalic veins, superior vena cava; ② the artery layer, the aorta and its three branches, right and left phrenic and vagus nerves; ③ the posterior layer, the trachea, esophagus, thoracic duct and left recurrent laryngeal nerve etc.

5.3.1   Thymus

It is the source of T lymphocytes which are associated with immune recognition. The thymus consists of two unequal later lobes connected by connective tissue. In fetus and infant, the thymus is large. It grows larger with ages, but after puberty it is gradually reduced and replaced by the connective tissue after mid-adult life.

5.3.2　Superior vena cava and its tributaries

The superior vena cava is converged by the right and left brachiocephalic veins behind the lower border of the right sternocostal synchondrosis of the 1st rib. It ends at the level of the lower border of the right 3rd sternocostal joint by entering into the right atrium. Before it pierces the pericardium, the azygos vein crosses over the root of the right lung and enter it.

Each of brachiocephalic vein is formed by the internal jugular and subclavian veins behind the corresponding sternoclavicular joint.

5.3.3　Aortic arch and its branches

The aortic arch is situated behind the lower half of the sternal manubrium. It continues with the ascending aorta behind the right second sternocostal joint, then arches from right and anterior to left and posterior and becomes the thoracic aorta to the left side of the lower border of the 4th thoracic vertebra. Its superior border is about at the level of midpoint of the sternal manubrium or slightly higher. On the convex aspect of the aortic arch, it gives off three branches from right to left: the brachiocephalic, the left common carotid artery and the left subclavian artery.

5.3.4　Arterial ligament

The arterial ligament is the arterial duct in fetus, and it becomes the ligament after birth. It connects the origin of the left pulmonary artery with the inferior surface of the end of aortic arch. The arterial ligament lies in the triangle of the ductus arteriosus which is formed by the left pulmonary artery inferiorly, the left phrenic nerve anteriorly and the left vagus nerve posteriorly.

5.3.5　The thoracic part of the trachea and the principal bronchi

The thoracic part of the trachea lies in the median plane of the posterior portion of the superior mediastinum, but it slightly deviates to the right in children. It bifurcates into the right and left principal bronchi approximately at the level of the sternal angle, but before one-year old, this bifurcation is higher, approximately at the level to the 3rd thoracic vertebra.

5.4　The inferior mediastinum

5.4.1　Anterior mediastinum

It contains the remains of the lower part of the thymus, the internal thoracic vessels and their branches, a part of the anterior mediastinal lymph nodes and some loose connective tissue.

5.4.2　Middle mediastinum

It contains the pericardium, the heart, and the roots of the great vessels from the heart, the arch of azygos vein, the phrenic nerves, the pericardiophrenic vessels, the cardiac plexuses and the lymph nodes.

● Pericardium   The pericardium consists of fibrous pericardium and serous pericardium. The fibrous pericardium, constituted by tough fibrous tissue is strong outer layer. Superiorly, it fused with adventitia of great blood vessels. Inferiorly, it is joined by the central tendon of the diaphragm. The serous pericardium is the internal layer which is transparent. The serous pericardium can be divided into parietal and visceral layers. The parietal layer lines the fibrous pericardium and is reflected around the roots of the great vessels to become continuous with the visceral layer. The visceral layer closely applied to the heart called the epicedium. The latent space between the parietal and visceral layers is called the pericardial cavity. Normally, the cavity contains a little serous fluid which lubricate or facilitate movements of the heart.

The sinuses of pericardium are formed by the irregular reflection of the parietal layer of the serous pericardium. They are the anteroinferior sinus, the oblique sinus and the transverse sinus.

● Blood supply in the pericardium   The roots of the great vessels within the pericardium are: ① the pulmonary trunk; ② the ascending aorta; ③ the superior vena cava; ④ the inferior vena cava; ⑤ the pulmonary veins.

● Heart   The heart, wrapped in the pericardium, rests its inferior surface on the central portion of the diaphragm, and its inferior border roughly corresponds to the level of the xiphisternal synchodrosis. Approximately one third of the heart lies to the right and two thirds to the left of the median plane.

Outline of the heart is commonly drawn by four points: ① The left superior point is 1.2 cm to the left border of the sternum at the level of the lower border of the 2nd rib on the left side. ② The right superior point is 1 cm to the right border of the sternum at the level of the upper border of the 3rd cartilage on the right side. ③ The right inferior point is at the 5th right sternocostal joint. ④ The left inferior point is 7-9 cm to the midline at the 5th left intercostal space.

5.5   The posterior mediastinum

It contains the following organs: the principal bronchi, thoracic part of the esophagus, thoracic aorta, thoracic duct, azygos and hemiazygos veins, vagus nerves, sympathetic trunks and lymph nodes.

5.5.1   The thoracic part of the esophagus

The thoracic part of the esophagus descends in front of the vertebral column in the superior and posterior mediastinum, passes through the esophageal hiatus of the diaphragm, and then become the abdominal part of the esophagus.

Anteriorly, the esophagus is adjacent to the trachea, left recurrent laryngeal nerve, left principal bronchus, pericardium and diaphragm. Posterior to the esophagus, there are the right posterior intercostal arteries, azygos and hemiazygos veins, the inferior part of the thoracic duct and the loose connective tissue. On the left side, the esophagus is adjacent to the left common carotid artery, left subclavian artery, aortic arch, thoracic aorta, the superior part of the thoracic duct, and the left mediastinal pleura, etc. On the right side, there are azygos vein and its arch, and right mediastinal pleura. Furthermore, the right and left vagus nerves descend along both sides of the esophagus at first, then give off the branches to form the esophagus plexus.

5.5.2　Thoracic aorta

The thoracic aorta continues with the aortic arch on the left side of the lower border of the 4th thoracic vertebra. It descends through the posterior mediastinum between the left pleura and the thoracic duct, the azygos vein. Lying posteriorly to the root of the left lung and then the pericardium, the thoracic aorta inclines to the right behind the esophagus to reach in front of the vertebral column and behind the diaphragm. At the anterior surface of the 12th thoracic vertabra, it passes through the aortic hiatus of the diaphragm to enter the abdominal cavity and becomes to the abdominal aorta.

The right surface of upper part of the thoracic aorta contacts with the esophagus, thoracic duct and azygos vein. The left surface is covered by the left mediastinal pleura. The lower part of the thoracic aorta lies right and posterior to the esophagus, right and anterior to the hemiazygos vein, left to the right mediastinal pleura, left and anterior to the thoracic duct.

5.5.3　Thoracic duct

The thoracic duct arises from the cisterna chyli in front of the 1st and 2nd lumbar vertebrae. It is formed by the union of the right and left lumbar trunks and the intestinal trunk. After it passes through the aortic hiatus of the diaphragm, the thoracic duct enter the posterior mediastinum against the right surface of the thoracic aorta. Between the thoracic aorta and the azygos vein, it ascends posterior to the esphagus. And then it gradually turns to the left of the median plane. At the level of the lower border of the 4th thoracic vertebra, the thoracic duct passes obliquely behind the esophagus to reach its left side, then ascends between the esophagus and the left pleura to the root of the neck.

5.5.4　The azygos, hemiazygos and accessory hemiazygos veins

The azygos vein arises from the right ascending lumbar vein in the abdomen, passes through the right crus of the diaphragm and enters the posterior. It runs upward on the anterior and right surfaces of the thoracic vertebrae, posterior and right to the thoracic aorta and esophagus. At the level of the 4th thoracic vertebra, it arches anteriorly and across the root of the right lung, then enters the superior vena cava. The hemiazygos vein begins with the left ascending lumbar vein, passes through the left crus of the diaphragm to enter the thoracic cavity. It ascends on the left side of the thoracic vertebrae, receives the left 8th to

11th posterior intercostal veins and left subcostal vein, then crosses the 8th thoracic verte-bra anteriorly to enter the azygos vein.

5.5.5　The thoracic part of the sympathetic trunk

The thoracic part of the sympathetic trunk consists of approximately $10 \sim 12$ ganglia on each side. The upper part of the trunk lie on the heads of ribs, and the lower part is lo-cated on the lateral surface of the vertebral bodies. The first thoracic ganglion is frequently fused with the inferior cervical ganglion to form the stellate ganglion before the neck of the 1st rib or the transverse process of the 7th ceivical vertebra. The ganglia communicates with the intercostal nerves by the white rami communicates and the grey rami communi-cates.

The upper four or five ganglia give off small branches to the esophageal, cardiac and pulmonary. The preganglionic fibers from the 8th to 10th thoracic segment of the spinal cord intermediolateral nucleus pass through the 5th to 9th ganglia to form the greater splanchnic nerve. The greater splanchnic nerve runs forward, pierces the crus of the dia-phragm and ends at the celiac ganglion in the abdominal cavity. The preganglionic fibers from the 10th to 12th thoracic segment of the spinal cord intermediolateral nucleus pass through the 10th to 12th ganglia to form the lesser splanchnic nerve which pierces the crus of the diaphragm and ends at the aorticoreanl ganglion.

5.5.6　Vagus nerves

In the thorax, to the left side of the aortic arch, the left vagus nerve runs downward between the left common carotid and subclavian arteries. On its way, the left vagus nerve gives off the left recurrent pharyngeal nerve which curves medially and rounds the inferior surface of the aortic arch posteriorly to the arterial ligament. And this recurrent paryngeal nerve ascends in the groove between the left side of the trachea and esophagus. The main trunk of the vagus nerve continually run downward behind the root of the left lung. The right vagus nerve descends posteriorly to the right surface of the trachea, posteriormedially to the superior vena cava, and posteriorly to the root of the right lung. The right recurrent pharygneal nerve encircles the anterior and inferior surfaces the right subclavian artery and ascends in the groove between the right side of the trachea and esophagus.

Behind the root of the lung, the two vagus nerves send branches to form the anterior and posterior pulmonary plexuses which enter the lung along the pricipal bronchi and pul-monaru vesels. The two vagus nerves also give off branches to form the esophageal plexus before and behind the esophagus. Finally, the two vagus nerves pierce the esophageal hia-tus accompanying the esophagus and enter the abdomen.

5.6　The mediastinal spaces

They are the narrow spaces among the organs in the mediastinum. The mediastinal spaces are filled with the loose connective tissue for adaptation of the changes of the organ's movement and bulk. It continues upward with the connective tissue and space of the neck, downward with the connective tissue and space of abdomen.

● Retrosternal space   It is between the sternum and the intrathoracic fascia.

● Pretracheal space   It is located among the trachea, the bifurcation of the trachea and the aortic arch within the superior mediastinum. Superiorly, it connects with the pretracheal space of the neck.

● Retroesophageal space   It is located between the esophagus and the intrathoracic fascia within the superior mediastinum. There are the thoracic duct, the azygos and the hemiazygos veins in the space. The retroesophageal space connects with the retroperitoneal space through the hiatus of the diaphragm.

Section 2
Dissection and observation

I. Thoracic wall and cavity

1　Position and incisions

The cadaver is placed in the supine position. Make skin incisions in the dissection of the pectoral region and axilla as follows:

● Make an incision in the midline from the suprasternal notch to xiphisternal junction.

● Make a curve incision along the costal margin to the midaxillary line.

● Make an oblique incision from the xiphisternal junction upward and laterally, around the nipple to the anterior axillary fold, then, along the medial side of the arm to the point between the upper and middle thirds.

2　Procedures

Examine the attachments of the pectoralis major, pectoralis minor and serratus anterior, the origins of the obliquus externus abdominis and rectus abdominis. Seek the anterior and lateral cutaneous branches of the intercostal nerves and the perforating branches of the internal thoracic vessels in two or three intercostal spaces.

Clean the digitations of the serratus anterior and the obliquus externus abdominis.

Strip the origin of the serratus anterior from the upper ribs and flip it laterally to the midaxillary line. The long thoracic nerve and lateral thoracic vessels on the surface of the serratus anterior. Remove the digitations of the obliquus externus abdominis to expose the ribs and the intercostales externi in 4th or 5th intercostal space.

Observe the intercostales externi in the 4th and 5th intercostal spaces Their fibers run from posterosuperior to anteroinferior. Anteriorly, the muscles are replaced by the external intercostal membrane. Then cut through the intercostales externi at anterolateral thoracic wall along the lower borders of the 4th and 5th ribs, and turn them downward to expose the intercostales interni, whose fibers are directed at right angles to the fibers of intercostales externi and pass downward and backward from the costal groove of the rib above to the superior border of the rib below.

Follow the lateral cutaneous branches of one or more intercostal nerves to the parent trunk deep to the intercostal muscles. Follow the trunk of the intercostal nerves. Follow the trunk of the intercostal nerves forward and backward with its accompanying vessels, cut away as much as of the lower margin of the intercostal muscles to expose the contents of the costal groove. Note the posterior intercostal artery and vein lie above the intercostal nerve. Follow the trunk of the intercostal nerves forward to find the anterior cutaneous branch. In the same intercostal space and along the superior margin of the lower rib, find the collateral branch of the posterior intercostal artery. The muscle which lies deep to the nerve and vessels is the intercostales intimi.

Remove the periosteum of the ribs and the intercostal muscles from 1st to 9th intercostal spaces between the anterior and posterior axillary lines. Take great care to protect the underlying pleura. Push away the parietal pleura from the thoracic wall.

Cut through the sternoclavicular joint or the middle part of the clavicle.

Cut through the 2nd to 10th ribs just posterior to the midaxillary line, cut through the 1st rib medial to the attachment of the scalenus anterior. Clean the remains of the muscles attached to the manubrium, push back the soft tissues from the manubrium, and find the internal thoracic artery in the 1st intercostal space and clean it. Then elevate the detached upper end of the anterior thoracic wall from the underlying structures by separating the ribs from the parietal pleura and the pericardium. Turn the anterior thoracic wall downward.

Observe the transversus thoracis, the internal thoracic vessels and its terminal branches, the superior epigastric and musculophrenic arteries on the inner surface of the anterior thoracic wall.

Remove the thymus or its remnants, observe the domes and anterior margins of the pleurae of both sides. The cupula (dome) of the pleura bulges up into the root of the neck. The anterior margins of the parietal pleurae of both sides converge as descend from the domes posterior to the sternoclavicular joints. They contact with each other between the level of the sternal angle and the level of the 4th costal cartilage. Between the level of the 4th and 6th costal cartilages, the anterior margin of the left parietal pleura deviates from the anterior midline and descends along the oblique line from the point of 2.5 cm lateral to the left border of the sternum to the midpoint of the 6th costal cartilage. Identify the triangle of pericardium behind the lower part of the sternal body, between the anterior borders of the pleurae on both sides.

Make a T-shaped incision in the anterior part of the parietal pleura opposite the 2nd to 6th ribs on each side. Explore the boundaries and extent of the pleural cavities, examine the costodiaphragmatic recess and costomediastinal recess. Remove the costal parietal pleura to expose the lung on each side, pull the lung laterally as much as possible to expose the root of the lung. Below the root of the lung, cut off the pulmonary ligament, then cut through the pulmonary root from upper downward close to the hilum of the lung in case of injuring the structures of the mediastinum and the lung. Identify the lobes of the lung, the structure passing through the hilum of the lung and their relationships.

On the inner surface of the posterior thoracic wall, strip the costal pleura of the 5th or 6th intercostal space carefully to expose the internal intercostal membrane lying medial to the angle of the ribs. Follow the internal intecostal membrane laterally to the fibers of the intercostales intimi. Cut off the intercostales intimi and expose the nerves and vessels with rum between the intercostales intimi and intercostales interni. Observe the course of the nerves and vessels.

Ⅱ. Lungs

1　Position

The cadaver is placed in the supine position.

2　Procedures

2.1　Observe the external feature of the lung

Each lung has an apex, two surfaces, three borders and a base. The apex of the lung projects into the root of neck. The surfaces are costal and medial surfaces. On the costal surface of the left lung, there is one oblique fissure that divides the left lung into superior and inferior lobes. On the right, oblique and horizontal fissure divide the right lung into superior, middle and inferior lobes. The borders are anterior, inferior and posterior borders. In the part of the anterior border of the left lung, there is a notch called the cardiac notch. The base is broad and concave, which accommodates the dome of the diaphragm.

2.2　Identify the structures in the root of lung

Examine the bronchus, pulmonary artery and pulmonary veins and the arrangement of them. The bronchus is located posteriorly, the pulmonary artery superiorly, and the pulmonary veins inferiorly. The right upper bronchus lies superiorly to the pulmonary artery.

Ⅲ. Mediastinum

1　Position

The cadaver is placed in the supine position.

2 Procedures

2.1 Strip the mediastinal pleura from both sides and observe the main structure around the root of the lungs

2.1.1 On the left side

Identify the structures surrounding the root of the left lung, they are: the aortic arch above, the left phrenic nerve and pericardiacophrenic vessels in front, and the thoracic aorta behind. The esophagus lies behind the left subclavian artery, where the esophagus slightly inclines to the left side. The thoracic duct clings to the left aspect of the esophagus. Behind the esophagus and the thoracic aorta, there are the thoracic part of the sympathetic trunk, thoracic sympathetic ganglia and greater splanchnic, descending on the left side of the thoracic vertebrae and lateral to the accessory hemiazygos and hemiazygos veins. The left vagus nerve lies to the left of the aortic arch and then runs downward between the root of the lung and the thoracic aorta. Under the root of the lung, between the pericardium and thoracic aorta, the esophagus appears to the right of the left vagus nerve.

2.1.2 On the right side

The azygos vein arches over the root of the right lung and enters the superior vena cava which enters the pericardium at the right side of the ascending aorta. The right phrenic nerve and pericardiacophrenic vessels lie before the root of the lung, and the right vagus nerve lies behind. Above the root of the lung, the trachea is situated behind the superior vena cava. Posterior to the right vagus nerve, from anterior to posterior, they are: the azygos vein, thoracic sympathetic trunk, thoracic sympathetic ganglia and greater splanchnic, descending on the right side of the thoracic vertebrae and lateral to the azygos vein.

2.2 Observe and identify the structures in the mediastinum

Find the thymus or its remnant, observe its size and lobes.

Remove the thymus and the connective tissue around it, and seek the lymph nodes along the inferior border of the left brachiocephalic vein. Identify the brachiocephalic vein and its tributaries which are the internal jugular vein, the subclavian vein, the vertebral vein, the internal thoracic vein, the inferior thyroid vein and some small veins in the upper intercostal spaces.

2.2.1 Clean and observe the ascending aorta

The aortic arch has three branches: the brachiocephalic trunk, the left common carotid artery and the left subclavian artery. Follow the aorta to the left side of the 4th thoracic vertebra where the aortic arch becomes the thoracic aorta. Identify the left phrenic and vagus nerves which pass left and anteriorly to the aortic arch and note the crossing of the two nerves above the aortic arch.

2.2.2   Follow and clean the pulmonary artery

The pulmonary (arterial) trunk arising from the right ventricle bifurcates into the right and left pulmonary arteries under the concavity of the aortic arch. Seek and clean the short, fibrous arterial ligament which connects the origin of the left pulmonary artery with the terminal part of the aortic arch.

2.2.3   Clean the right phrenic and vagus nerves

The right phrenic nerve enters the thoracic cavity between the subclavian artery and vein, then it passes in front of the root of the lung accompanying the pericardiacophrenic vessels to the diaphragm. Between the right subclavian artery and vein, look for the right vagus nerve which descends on the right of the trachea, posteromedial to the right brachiocephalic vein and the superior vena cava, then passes behind the root of the right lung to approach the right and posterior surface of the esophagus.

Cut off the left brachiocephalic vein and turn it upward. Pull the brachiocephalic trunk and left common carotid artery laterally, trace and clean the thoracic part of the trachea and the right and left principal bronchi. Look for the paratracheal lymph nodes and the tracheobronchial lymph nodes.

2.2.4   Observe the pericardium

Make a vertical incision on each side of the pericardium immediately anterior the phrenic nerve to the transverse incision 2 cm above the diaphragm. Strip the flap upward to examine the pericardial cavity and the pericardial sinus. Observe the anteroinferior sinus lying between the anterior and inferior walls of the pericardium.

2.2.5   Observe the sinus of pericurdium

Insert a finger or a forceps between the ascending aorta and the lowest part of the superior vena cava, push it to the left and the finger or the forceps move between the pulmonary trunk and the left auricle. The space where the finger or forceps stay is called the transverse sinus of the pericardium. Lift the heart from the diaphragmatic pericardium and insert a finger superiorly behind the heart to explore the space that lies among the right and left pulmonary veins, superior vena cava, the left atrium and the posterior wall of the parietal pericardium.

2.2.6   Clean and trace the thoracic aorta

The thoracic aorta continues with the aortic arch and begins at the level of the lower border of the 4th thoracic vertebra left to the vertebral column. Then it descends along the left side of the vertebral bodies of 5th, 6th and 7th thoracic vertebrae and turns in front of the vertebral bodies of the lower four thoracic vertebrae. Before the body of the thoracic vertebra, it lies behind the esophagus. At the level of the 12th thoracic vertebra, it passes through the aortic hiatus of the diaphragm and enters the abdomen. At its course, the thoracic aorta gives off the posterior intercostal arteries and subcostal arteries.

Look for the left recurrent laryngeal nerve in the left groove between the trachea and the esophagus, and trace it downward to the aortic arch, upward to the neck.

Clean and observe the hemiazygos and accessory hemiazygos veins on the left side of the thoracic vertebra and trace them to where they enter the azygos vein or the hemiazygos vein.

Seek the lower part of the thoracic duct between the azygos vein and the thoracic aorta. Trace it upward and identify its course and relationships. It ascends obliquely behind the esophagus to reach the left side at the level of the 4th intervertebral disc.

On the right side of the thoracic, clean the azygos vein and observe it. Clean the esophagus and identify its relationships.

Strip the connective tissue on each side of the thoracic vertebrae, observe the thoracic part of the sympathetic trunk, thoracic ganglia and communicating branches between the sympathetic trunk and intercostal nerves. Examine the great splanchnic nerve formed by the branches arising from the 5th to 9th sympathetic ganglia.

Strip the parietal pleura and connective tissue on the posterior thoracic wall, clean the intercostal nerve and vessels and observe the arrangement of them.

Section 3

Clinical application

I. Breast cancer

The breast cancer is commonly found at the upper outer quadrant(or the axillary tail). The pectoralis major, pectoralis minor, and the lymph nodes in the axillary cavity must be widely excised in radical mastectomy. When cleaning the pectoral lymph nodes, the long thoracic nerve on the serratus anterior must not be damaged. When cleaning the lymph nodes of the lateral and central groups, the vessels and nerves, especially the axillary vein ought to be protected and saved. When removing the lymph nodes of the apical group, the cephalic vein must be separated and retained.

II. Pleuracentesis

In a patient with pleuracentesis, any fluid accumulated in the pleural cavity can be drained by inserting a needle through an intercostal space (usually the 7th or 8th on the posterior axillary line). The needle must be inserted along the superior border of the lower rib in case of injuring the intercostal nerve and vessels. Below the 8 th intercostal space, the diaphragm is likely to be injured.

III. Pleura

The visceral pleura is insensitive to pain, while the parietal pleura is very sensitive to pain, particularly its costal part. Irritation of the costal and peripheral diaphragm areas results in local pain and also in referred pain along the intercostal nerves to the thoracic and abdominal wall, whereas irritation of the mediastinal and central diaphragmatic areas results in referred pain in the lower part of the neck and over the shoulder.

IV. Constrictions of the esophagus

The upper constriction of the esophagus is its commencement at the end of the pharynx in the neck. The middle constriction lies behind the left principal bronchus. The lower constriction is the part passing through the esophageal hiatus. These constrictions may be observed as narrowing of the lumen in oblique radiographs with swallowing barium as a marker. These constrictions are common site of carcinoma of esophagus, and they are also prone to hide the foreign bodies or foods in the esophagus.

V. Diaphragm

The diaphragm serves as a portion between the cavities of thorax and abdomen. Imperfect development, weakness, or injury to the diaphragm may permit abdominal viscera to protrude into the thoracic cavity (diaphragmatic hernia).

Section 4

Ask yourself

1. In the costal groove, what is the arrangement of the intercostal nerve and vessels?

2. Explain the lymphatic drainage of the female breast.

3. Explain the pleura and pleural cavity.

4. What are the main structures in the root of the right lung? What is the arrangement of them from the top downward?

5. Explain the divisions of the mediastinum.

6. What are the structures in superior mediastinum?

7. Describe the pericardium and pericardial cavity.

8. What are the openings of the diaphragm? What structure pass through the openings respectively?

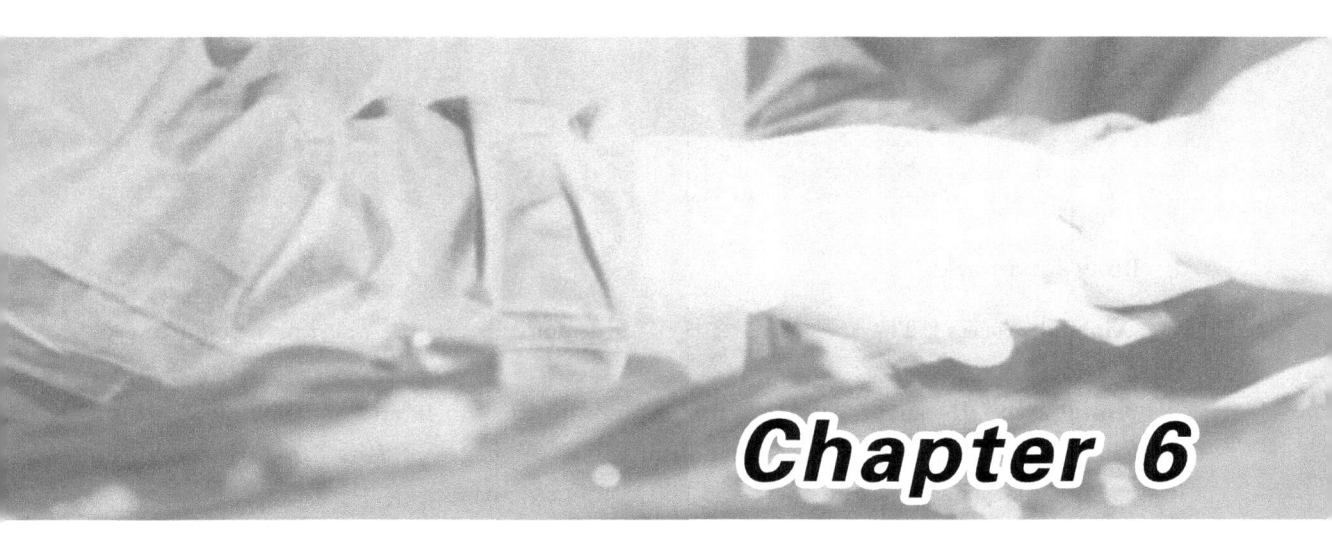

Chapter 6

The abdomen

Section 1

Review

Ⅰ. Surface anatomy

1 Bony landmarks

Xiphoid process   The lowest part of the sternum, lies in the anterior median line of the body.

Costal arch   It can be palpated from xiphoid process to lateral and oblique down on both sides. It is formed by the connection of costal cartilages of 7th, 8th, 9th and 10th. It's the boundary between the chest and belly on body surface.

Iliac crest and anterior superior iliac spine   The superior border of ilium (iliac ala) is iliac crest which can be touched on both sides of lower part of abdomen. The anterior round end of it is anterior superior iliac spine which can be easily palpated in living body. The highest part of the iliac crest is called the iliac tubercle, the line connected both sides of them passes through the spine of 4th lumbar vertebra horizontally.

Pubic symphysis and pubic tubercle   The pubic symphysis is a conjunction area of right and left hip bones in front at the lowest part of abdomen, can be touched from umbilicus downward. The pubic tubercle is lateral to pubic symphysis.

2 Muscular landmarks

Linea alba   It locates on the middle line of the abdomen and between the left and right rectus sheath attaching to xiphoid process superiorly and pubic symphysis inferiorly, formed by interwoven fibers of the rectus sheath on both sides. This line is wider above the umbilicus and narrower below, there is a circular ring at midpoint of it, termed umbilical ring.

Semilunar line   The lateral border of the rectus muscles, curved convex laterally, from the pubic tubercle up to the tip of 9th costal cartilage.

Umbilicus   It lies on anterior median abdominal line at the level of the 3th～4th intervertebral disc.

Inguinal ligament   There is a groove between the thigh and the abdomen, inguinal groove, the boundary between them. The inguinal ligament is deep to it, attaches to the pubic tubercle and anterior superior iliac spine.

II . Boundaries and divisions

The abdomen lies at the lower part of the trunk between the thorax and the pelvis. Its boundaries superiorly is formed by the xiphoid process midpoint and costal arches both sides; inferiorly by the line connects pubic symphysis, pubic crests, pubic tubercles, inguinal grooves, anterior superior iliac spines and iliac crests each other on the body surface. Inside of the trunk, the abdominal cavity is separated to the thoracic cavity by the diaphragm above; communicated with pelvic cavity below.

There are nine regions of the abdomen divided by two transverse and two sagittal planes. The upper transverse plane passes through the lowest points of the costal arches, the lower one passes though the crest tubercles. The sagittal planes run though the midpoint of the inguinal ligament or the clavicle each side.

Table 6 – 1   The surface projections of the visceral organs

right hypochondriac region	epigastric region	left hypochondriac region
right lobe of the liver gallbladder right colic flexure right kidney right suprarenal gland	left lobe of the liver little part of the stomach upper part of the duodenum head and body of pancreas common bile duct	left lobe of the liver large part of the stomach tail of the pancreas spleen and left kidney left suprarenal gland left colic flexure
right lateral region	**umbilical region**	**left lateral region**
ascending colon ileum lower part of kidney	transverse colon great omentum small intestine ureters	descending colon jejunum lower part of kidney
right inguinal region	**hypogastric region**	**left inguinal region**
ending of ileum cecum vermiform appendix	jejunum and ileum urinary bladder(fill up) uterus(pregnant) ureters	ileum sigmoid colon

III. Main contents

1 Anteriolateral abdominal wall

1.1 Layers from superficial to deep

1.1.1 Skin

It's thin and elastic, the mobility of the groin area is little and the skin flaps with vessels is used for plastic surgery commonly.

1.1.2 Superficial fascia

There is only one layer above the umbilical plane. Below the umbilicus, it is divided into two layers as below:

Superficial layer (fat layer)—Camper's fascia, with more adipose tissue, it is continuous with the superficial fascia of the thigh downward and back, which is thicker in the inguinal region.

Deep layer(membranous layer) Scarpa's fascia, rich in elastic fibers, is attached to the white line in the midline; continued to the fascia lata of the thigh below the inguinal ligament about one finger width; continued to the superficial perineal fascia (fascia of Colles) of the scrotum below the level of pubic tubercle.

The superficial epigastric artery, the superficial circumflex iliac artery and the accompanying veins run between them.

▶ Superficial arteries

Upper part—originate from the branches of 7th ～11th pairs of the posterior intercostal arteries, subcostal artery and lumbar arteries lateral side, and superior epigastric artery medial side.

Lower part—originate from the superficial epigastric artery and the superficial iliac circumflex artery arising from the femoral artery. They are mostly used to the pedicled skin flap in clinic.

▶ Superficial veins

The venous anastomoses are rich especially in the umbilical area.

Above the umbilicus—drains into the axillary vein passing through the superficial thoracoepigastric vein.

Umbilical area—runs into the hepatic portal vein passing through the paraumbilical vein surrounding the umbilical cord inwards.

Below the umbilicus—drains into the great saphenous vein passing through the superficial epigastric vein and the superficial circumflex iliac vein.

So, the periumbilical venous rete is the anastomoses between the superior vena cava and inferior vena cava, the vena cava with the hepatic portal vein.

▶ Superficial lymph

It drains to the axillary lymph nodes above the level of umbilicus.

It drains to the superficial inguinal lymph nodes below the umbilicus.

▶ Cutaneous nerve

It comes from the lower part of intercostal nerves, subcostal nerve, iliohypogastric nerve and the ilioinguinal nerve (T7~L1).

The 7th intercostal nerve distributes in the area just a little lower under the level of the xiphoid process; the 10th intercostal nerve in the area of level of the umbilicus; the L1 lumbar nerve in the area just above the inguinal ligament.

1.1.3 Deep fascia

It's very thin that can be ignored.

1.1.4 Muscles

The muscles can be subdivided into anteriolateral group and posterior group.

● Anteriolateral group

Rectus abdominis is long strip-like, it lies from anterior lower thoracic cage to the pubic crest.

Externus obliquus abdominis originates from external surface and the inferior borders of the lower 8 ribs. Its fiber runs downward and medially changes into aponeurosis. Between the pubic tubercle and anterior superior iliac spine, its aponeurosis forms the inguinal ligament, some fibers of its medial end are attached to the pubic pectin as the lacunar ligament, other parts are reflected to the rectus sheath and linea alba as the reflected ligament. The aponeurosis near pubic tubercle forms the superficial inguinal ring and the external spermatic fascia.

Internus obliquus abdominis, its fibers arise from the lateral 2/3 of the inguinal ligament, the iliac crest and the thoracolumbar fascia, run upward and medially. The lowest part fibers run over the spermatic cord and join in the inguinal falx (conjoined tendon) and the cremaster.

Transversus abdominis is innermost, it arises from the lateral 1/3 of the inguinal ligament, the iliac crest, the thoracolumbar fascia and the internal surface of lower 6 costal cartilages. Its fibers go medially, the lowest part fibers join in with the internus obliquus abdominis.

The aponeurosis of three layers flat muscles form the semilunar line, the rectus sheath and the linea alba.

● Posterior group On the posterior wall of abdomen is the quadratus lumborum.

1.1.5 Deep vessels and nerves

There are the 7th~11th intercostal nerves, subcostal nerve and their accompanying arteries and veins; superior and inferior epigastric arteries and veins supply deep structures.

1.1.6 Transverse fascia

It's a thin layer between the extraperitoneal fascia and the transverse abdominis. It is thick in the inguinal region, and it forms the deep inguinal ring and the internal spermatic fascia.

1.1.7 Extraperitoneal fascia (extraperitoneal fatty tissue)

It's a layer of loose connective tissue with fat between the transverse fascia and the parietal peritoneum, can be considered as a space, termed extraperitoneal space.

1.1.8 Parietal peritoneum

It is the innermost layer of the abdominal wall, there are several peritoneal folds and fossae at lower part.

1.2 Rectus sheath

It's formed by three layers aponeuroses. There is a plane at about 4 cm below the umbilicus (the arcuate line). The arcuate line is lower free margin of the posterior rectus sheath.

Above arcuate line, the anterior sheath is formed by the aponeurosis of externus obliquus abdominis and anterior layer aponeurosis of internus obliquus abdominis; the posterior sheath is formed by the aponeurosis of transversus abdominis and posterior layer of aponeurosis of internus obliquus abdominis.

Below arcuate line, the anterior sheath is formed by all three layers of aponeuroses, the posterior sheath is lack.

1.3 Inguinal region

A weak area of inferior part of the anterior abdominal wall, which is the anatomical basis of the hernias and hydrocele.

1.3.1 Inguinal canal

It lies just above the medial half of the inguinal ligament one finger width, is a potential cleft about 4 cm long in the muscles.

▶ Two openings

The superficial inguinal ring (external inguinal opening) is a triangular opening in shape of the externus obliquus abdominis superiolateral to the pubic tubercle.

The deep inguinal ring(internal inguinal opening) is an a entrance of inguinal canal at the midpoint of the inguinal ligament just above one finger breadth and is formed by the transverse fascia.

▶ Four walls

The anterior wall is formed by the aponeurosis of externus obliquus abdominis and enforced by internal oblique muscle of abdomen laterally.

The posterior wall is formed by the transverse fascia and enforced by inguinal falx and reflected ligament medially.

The superior wall is formed by the inferior arcuate fibers of internus obliquus abdominis and transversus abdominis.

The inferior wall is formed by medial half of the inguinal ligament.

▶ Contents

The spermatic cord (in the male) or the round ligament of uterus (in the female) and the ilioinguinal nerve pass though it.

1.3.2 Inguinal triangle (Hesslbach's triangle)

It is located in the medial part of inguinal region, medially bounded by the lateral border of rectus abdominis, inferiorly by medial half of the inguinal ligament and laterally by the inferior epigastric vessels.

2 Peritoneum and peritoneal cavity

The peritoneum attaches on the inner surface of the abdominal and pelvic walls and the surface of most internal organs, which is smooth. The lining in inner surface of the abdominal and the pelvic wall is called parietal peritoneum; coated on the organ surface is the visceral peritoneum. The peritoneal cavity is a latent space between that two continuous parts. The peritoneal cavity is confined in the male while it is open to the outside through reproductive ducts in the female.

2.1 The structures formed by the peritoneum

2.1.1 Omenta

● Lesser omentum It's a double layers peritoneal fold extended from the inferior surface of liver (porta hepatis) to the lesser curvature of stomach and upper part of the duodenum. It is divided into hepatogastric ligament left larger part and hepatoduodenal ligament right smaller part. The right free margin of the lesser omentum (hepatoduodenal ligament) contains the common bile duct (right anterior), the proper hepatic artery (left anterior) and the hepatic portal vein (behind).

● Greater omentum It's a four layers peritoneal fold hanging down from the stomach and the transverse colon. The anterior two layers which descend from the greater curvature of stomach and commencement of the duodenum pass downward in front of the small intestine for a variable distance; then they fold on themselves and ascend as far as the transverse colon. The lower part of greater omentum is adherent for a different extent, between the greater curvature of the stomach and the transverse colon, it is referred to as the gastrocolic ligament.

● Omental (epiploic) foramen It's called the foramen Winslow, which lies behind the right free margin of the lesser omentum, communicates the omental bursa to the greater peritoneal sac. It's bounded by the hepatoduodenal ligament in front, inferior vena cava behind, caudate lobe of the liver above, upper part of the duodenum below.

● Omental bursa It locates behind the lesser omentum and the stomach, bounded by

Anteriorly: the lesser omentum, the posterior wall of the stomach, the anterior two layers of the greater omentum.

Posteriorly: the posterior two layers of the greater omentum, the transverse colon and its mesocolon, the peritoneum covering the pancreas and left kidney.

Superiorly: the inferior surface of caudate lobe of the liver and the peritoneum covering the diaphragm.

Inferiorly: the reflected area of the anterior and posterior two layers of the greater omentum or the gastrocolic ligament.

Left: the spleen, the gastrosplenic and the splenorenal ligaments.

Right: opens to the greater peritoneal sac through the omental foramen.

2.1.2 Mesenteries

It's two layers of peritoneum, there is the role of fixation for organs such as mesostenium, mesoappendix, transverse mesocolon and sigmoid mesocolon.

● Mesentery of small intestine (or mesostenium) It's a broad, fan-shaped peritoneal fold connecting the jejunum and ileum to the posterior abdominal wall. The root of the mesentery is about 15 cm long and extends downward obliquely from the duodenojejunal flexure to the upper part of the right sacroiliac joint. It contains the superior mesenteric vessels, lymph nodes, nerve and some fat.

● Mesoappendix It is a triangular peritoneal fold which attached to the back of the lower end of the mesentery and close to the vermiform appendix.

● Transverse mesocolon It is a broad peritoneal fold which connects the transverse colon to the posterior abdominal wall, in front of the head and body of the pancreas.

● Sigmoid mesocolon It is a fold of the peritoneum which attaches the sigmoid colon to the pelvic wall. The sigmoid and superior rectal vessels run in it.

2.1.3 Ligaments

They are peritoneal folds formed by the transitional part of peritoneum, from the body wall to the viscera or from one organ to another, that there is a certain fixed function to the organs. Such as the falciform ligament and coronary ligament, triangular ligament of liver, the hepatoduodenal ligament and hepatogastric ligament, the gastrolienal ligament, gastrophrenic ligament, gastropancreatic ligament, gastrocolic ligament of the stomach, lienorenal ligament, phrenicosplenic ligament, the broad ligament of the uterus etc.

2.1.4 Recesses

● Superior and inferior duodenal recesses

● Superior and inferior ileocecal recesses

● Retrocecal recess

● Intersigmoid recess

2.1.5　Pouches

In the lesser pelvis, the peritoneum dips downward forming a large fossa, named the pouch. In the male, there is a rectovesical pouch between the rectum and urinary bladder. In the female, the uterus and its broad ligament divide the pouches.

2.1.6　Folds

There are 5 folds of the parietal peritoneum on the lower part of anterior abdominal wall.

2.2　Divisions of the peritoneal cavity

The peritoneal cavity is subdivided by the transverse colon and its mesocolon.

● Supracolic compartment　It lies between the diaphragm and the transverse mesocolon which contains the liver, gallbladder, stomach, spleen, pancreas, duodenum and their vessels, nerves, lymph.

● Infracolic compartment　It lies below the transverse mesocolon. It contains the jejunum, ileum, cecum, vermiform appendix, colon and their mesenteries, vessels, nerves and lymph.

● Retroperitoneal space　It lies behind the peritoneum covering the posterior abdominal wall. It contains the kidney, suprarenal gland, ureter, abdominal aorta and it's branches, inferior vena cava and it's tributaries, sympathetic trunk, etc.

3　The supracolic compartment

3.1　Anatomy of the abdominal esophagus

The abdominal esophagus, which is $1\sim2$ cm long, starts at the level of the esophageal hiatus of diaphragm and connects to the cardia of stomach. It is related to the left lobe of liver anteriorly, and the left crus of diaphragm posteriorly. The left and right vagi lie on its anterior and posterior surface respectively.

It's supplied by the branches from the left gastric artery; the veins drain into the left gastric vein, and then to the hepatic portal vein.

About the lymphatic drainage and nerve supplying, please refer the textbook.

3.2　Anatomy of the stomach

3.2.1　Position and relations

Locates in the left hypochondriac region mostly, a small part in the epigastric region about moderate gastric filling. The cardia is on the left side of the 11th thoracic vertebra, the pylorus is on the right side of the 1st lumbar vertebra.

The anterior wall of the stomach on the right side is related to the left lobe of liver;

left upper portion to the diaphragm and the lower portion to the anterior abdominal wall. The posterior wall of stomach contacts with the stomach bed (the diaphragm, left suprarenal gland, left kidney, pancreas, spleen, transverse colon and its mesocolon) by omental bursa.

3.2.2 Ligaments

There are the gastrohepatic ligament, gastrocolic ligament, gastrosplenic ligament and gastrophrenic ligament. The gastrosplenic ligament runs from upper part of the greater curvature to the hilum of spleen; the gastrophrenic ligament runs from the fundus of stomach to the diaphragm.

3.2.3 Blood supply

● Arteries   They all origin from the celiac trunk.

The left gastric artery originates from the celiac trunk, near to the right side of cardia, runs along the lesser curvature of the stomach to the right side.

The right gastric artery originates from the proper hepatic artery, descending to the pylorus and runs along the lesser curvature of the stomach to the left side.

These two arteries between the two layer of lesser omentum near the edge of the lesser curvature anatomizes arterial arch, branch to anterior and posterior wall of the stomach.

The right gastroepiploic artery originates from the gastroduodenal artery, between the anterior two layers of greater omentum runs along the greater curvature of the stomach to left side.

The left gastroepiploic artery originates from the splenic artery in the gastrosplenic ligament, along the greater curvature of the stomach to right side between the anterior two layers of the greater omentum.

These two arteries join each other and form arterial arch, they distribute to the greater curvature of the stomach and greater omentum.

The short gastric artery originates from the end of the splenic artery or its branches to the fundus of stomach in the gastrosplenic ligament.

The posterior gastric artery it is about 72%, originates from the splenic artery, to the posterior wall of omental bursa and the posterior wall of the gastric fundus.

● Veins   Accompany with the same name arteries, drain into the hepatic portal vein finally.

The right and left gastric veins drain into the hepatic portal vein directly; the short gastric vein, posterior gastric vein and left gastroepiploic vein drain into the splenic vein, and then to the hepatic portal vein; the right gastroepiploic vein enters into the superior mesenteric vein, and then to the hepatic portal vein.

3.2.4 Lymphatic drainage

● Left and right gastric lymph nodes   The lymph nodes distribute to the the corre-

Chapter 6 The abdomen

sponding area of the anterior and posterior walls of the stomach and arranged along the blood vessel.

- Left and right gastroepiploic lymph nodes   The arrangement lies along the greater curvature of the corresponding vessels.
- Cardiac lymph node
- Superior and inferior pyloric lymph nodes
- Splenic lymph nodes   All of the efferent lymphatic ducts drain into the celiac lymph node.

3.2.5   Innervation

It is supplied by autonomic nerves.

- Motor fibers   The preganglionic sympathetic nerve comes from T6～T10 in the greater splanchnic nerve, make relay in the celiac ganglion, the postganglionic fibers to the stomach wall and inhibit gastric peristalsis and reduce gastric acid secretion; the preganglionic parasympathetic nerve coming from the vagus nerve (anterior vagal trunk-anterior gastric branches; posterior vagal trunk-posterior gastric branches) is to enhance gastric peristalsis and gastric acid secretion.

- Sensory fibers   They run within the sympathetic and parasympathetic nerve to the spinal cord and medulla.

3.3   Anatomy of the duodenum

Duodenum is the initial part of the small intestine, which is about 20～25 cm long. The upper end connects to the pylorus of the stomach and the lower connects with the jejunum at duodenojejunal flexure. The duodenum bends like "C" shaped, wrapped around the head of the pancreas. In addition to the both ends, it is extraperitoneal.

3.3.1   Portions and relations

There are four parts according to its course.

Upper part—about 4～5 cm long, anteriosuperior is related to the quadrate lobe of liver and gallbladder, inferior is adjacent to the head of pancreas; the common bile duct, gastroduodenal artery and vein, hepatic portal vein and inferior vena cava behind it.

Descending part—about 7～8 cm long, lies right side of 1～3 lumbar vertebrae. The transverse colon and mesocolon Pass through it in front, the right lobe of the liver and small intestine loop is adjacent to superior and inferior respectively; the right renal hilum and the origin of the ureter adjacent to posteriorly; the pancreatic head and the common bile duct medially, the right colic flexure adjacent to laterally.

Transverse part—about 10～20 cm long, crossing the 3rd lumbar vertebra in front to the left. The superior is adjacent to the head of the pancreas; the anterior to the loop of small intestine, root of mesentery and the superior mesenteric vessels; the posterior to the right ureter, inferior vena cava, abdominal aorta and spine.

— 123 —

Ascending part—about 2~3 cm long, runs up to the left side of 2nd lumbar vertebra, continues to the jejunum with the duodenojejunal flexure. Right side of it is related to the head of pancreas and the aorta.

3.3.2 Suspensory ligament

Also known as the Treitz ligament, which is composed by fibrous and muscular tissue, from the duodenojejunal flexure up to the right crus of diaphragm. It can fix the duodenum.

3.3.3 Blood supply

There are the superioanterior and superioposterior pancreaticoduodenal artery, inferior pancreaticoduodenal artery mainly, from the gastroduodenal artery and superior mesenteric artery respectively.

The corresponding veins enter into the hepatic portal vein finally.

3.4 Anatomy of the liver

3.4.1 Position and relations

Most of the liver lies in the right hypochondriac and epigastric region, a small part in the left hypochondriac region. Except in the epigastric area, the rest of liver is covered by ribs and costal cartilages. The lower edge of the liver in children was lower than the costal arch but within 2 cm, which could not be reached after 7 years old.

The diaphragmatic surface of the liver is adjacent to the diaphragm which separates it from right pleural cavity, right lung and pericardium. The visceral surface of right lobe contact with the right kidney, right colic flexure and upper part of duodenum, left lobe with the stomach and esophagus.

3.4.2 Ligaments

There are falciform ligament, coronary and triangular ligaments on the anterior and superior surface of liver attaching to anterior abdominal wall and diaphragm respectively; the right and left triangular ligaments are the free margins of both ends of coronary ligaments. The bare area of liver lies at the posterosuperior of the liver, between both layers of coronary ligament, that is fixed to diaphragm by connective tissue. The round ligament of liver, closed umbilical vein, lies in lower border of the falciform ligament. The hepatogastric and hepatoduodenal ligaments also have a role of fixation for the liver.

3.4.3 Porta hepatis and hepatic pedicle

There is a "H" shaped deep groove on the visceral surface of liver: the left and right longitudinal grooves, transverse groove. The transverse groove lies between the left and the right longitudinal grooves is called porta hepatis or the first porta hepatis. The left and right branches of the proper hepatic artery, the left and right branches of the hepatic portal vein and the left and right hepatic ducts leave or enter the liver mainly.

The left, middle and right hepatic veins drain into inferior vena cava in the upper part of the fossa of vena cava, the second porta hepatis.

Some small veins from the right and caudate lobe of liver drain into inferior vena cava in the lower part of the fossa of vena cava, the third porta hepatis.

The hepatic artery and its branches, hepatic duct, portal vein and its branches, lymphatic vessels and nerves, are common within the connective tissue, called hepatic pedicle. Arrangement of main structures of the hepatic pedicle, is left and right hepatic ducts, left and right hepatic arteries, left and right branches of hepatic portal vein anterioposteriorly.

3.4.4 Lobes and segment

Please refer the textbook.

3.4.5 Blood supply, lymphatic drainage and innervation

The blood supply of liver comes from the proper hepatic artery and hepatic portal vein. The former occupies 30%, mainly oxygen; the latter occupies 70%, mainly nutrients from gastrointestine tract. The venous blood of liver enter into the inferior vena cava.

The lymph of the liver drains into the hepatic lymph nodes and posteriormediastinal lymph nodes through the superior and deep lymphatic vessels of the liver finally.

The nerves of the liver contain sympathetic and parasympathetic fibers reaching the liver by the way of hepatic plexus from the celiac plexus.

3.5 Anatomy of extrahepatic bile duct

It is composed of the left and right hepatic ducts, common hepatic duct, common bile duct and gall bladder, etc.

3.5.1 The gallbladder

The gallbladder is located in the gallbladder fossa on inferior surface of the liver. It can be divided into four parts: the fundus, the body, the neck and the cystic duct. The fundus of gallbladder projects below the inferior border of the liver and is adjacent to the posterior surface of anterior abdominal wall, near the tip of 9th right costal cartilage, where the lateral border of right rectus abdominis (or right midclavicular line) crosses to the right costal arch. The body of gallbladder lies in the fossa, the neck of gallbladder is continuous with the body at the right end of the porta hepatic and forms a S-shaped curve to join the cystic duct.

▶ Relations

Superiorly, the gallbladder relates to the liver; inferiorly andposteriorly, the superior part of the duodenum and the transverse colon; anteriorly, the anterior abdominal wall; left side, the pylorus; right side, the right colic flexure.

The cystic duct is continuous with neck of gallbladder, and then passes downward, backward, and to the left and runs parallel to the common hepatic duct before joining it. For the variations of the cystic duct, please refer the textbook.

▶ Blood vessels, lymphatic drainage and innervation

The cystic artery is often in the triangle of Calot starting from the right hepatic artery (the right branch of the proper hepatic artery). This triangle is bordered by the cystic duct, the common hepatic duct and inferior surface of the liver. About the variations of the cystic artery, please refer the textbook. The cystic vein drains into the hepatic portal vein.

The lymph of the gallbladder drains into the hepatic lymph nodes.

The nerve of the gallbladder is supplied by the hepatic plexus from the celiac plexus. It also receives the nerve fiber from the right phrenic nerve.

3.5.2　Bile duct

The common bile duct is formed by the union of the cystic duct and common hepatic duct (the union by the left and right hepatic ducts). It is about $0.6\sim0.8$ cm in diameter and $7\sim8$ cm in length, and it can be divided into four segments.

Supraduodenal part (first segment) goes down in the free margin of the hepatoduodenal ligament, right side of the proper hepatic artery and in front of the hepatic portal vein. This part of duct can be palpated by putting a finger into the omental foramen.

Retroduodenal part (second segment) goes down behind the upper part of the duodenum, the inferior vena cava lies posteriorly, the hepatic portal vein and gastroduodenal artery lies in the left side.

Pancreatic part (third segment) runs downward in the groove or is embedded in the posterior surface of head of pancreas in front of the inferior vena cava.

Introduodenal part (fourth segment) is just $1.5\sim2$ cm long. It passes the posteriomedial wall of descending duodenum obliquely, forms hepatopancreatic ampulla(Vater ampulla), the union with the pancreatic duct, opens in the major duodenal papilla, about $7.5\sim10$ cm from the pylorus.

The thickened circular muscles around the lower part of the common bile duct and the terminal part of pancreatic duct is called the sphincter of hepatopancreatic ampulla (or the sphincter of Oddi). Please refer the textbook for details.

3.6　Anatomy of the pancreas

The pancreas has head, neck, body and tail from right to left.

3.6.1　Position and relations

It lies in the epigastric and left hypochondriac regions, at the level of the 1st and 2nd lumber vertebrae, and behind the peritoneum on the posterior abdominal wall.

The head of pancreas is surrounded by the C-shaped duodenum. The common bile duct is behind the upper lateral part of it or sometimes runs within it. The inferior vena cava and right renal vein is posterior to it. The root of transverse mesocolon is in front of it.

The neck of pancreas is a narrow slender part between the head and body of pancreas. The superior mesenteric vein and the beginning of narrower comparing with the hepatic portal vein is behind it, the pylorus is anteriorsuperior to it.

The body of pancreas is longer and in front of spine. It aparted with the posterior wall of stomach by the omental bursa; posteriorly, it faces the abdominal aorta, left suprarenal gland, left kidney and splenic vein. The splenic artery runs just above upper border of it.

The tail of pancreas lies within the splenorenal ligament, the tip of it touches the hilum of spleen. It is related to the left colic flexure inferiorly, to the left kidney and suprarenal gland posterior.

3.6.2 Pancreatic ducts and its opening

The main pancreatic duct starts from the tail of pancreas tail and runs up to the right in the body to head. Along its course, it receives small tributaries, unites with the common bile duct finally, and then opens to the major duodenal papilla together.

3.6.3 Blood supply, lymphatic drainage and innervation

Please refer the textbook for details.

3.7 Anatomy of the spleen

3.7.1 Position and relations

The spleen is situated in the left hypochondriac region of abdomen. It lies obliquely with its long axis and parallels with the 9th, 10th, and 11th ribs. Normally, it couldn't be palpated below the costal arch.

The diaphragmatic surface face the diaphragm; the visceral surface is adjacent to the stomach, left kidney, left colic flexure and tail of pancreas.

3.7.2 Ligament

The spleen is a intraperitoneal organ. The peritoneum that surrounds it and connects with others forms several ligaments as follow: gastrosplenic ligament, phrenicosplenic ligament and splenorenal ligament.

3.7.3 Blood supply, lymphatic drainage and innervation

Please refer the textbook for details.

4 Infracolic compartment

4.1 The anatomy of jejunum and ileum

4.1.1 Position

The jejunum and ileum are the continuous coiled part of the small intestine. The jejunum occupies the upper 2/5 and locates in the upper left abdominal cavity near to the umbilical region. The ileum occupies lower 3/5 and lies in the lower right abdominal cavity near to the hypogastric region.

4.1.2 Mesentery

It is a double layers structure of peritoneum, and contains the jejunal and ileal blood vessels, nerves, lymphatics, lymph nodes and some fat. The root of mesentery begins from the duodenojejunal flexure at the left side of 2nd lumbar vertebra, it then extends obliquely downward and ends to the ileocecal junction at the level of the right sacroiliac joint approximately.

4.1.3　Blood supply, lymphatic drainage and innervation

They are supplied by several jejunal and ileal arteries originating from the superior mesenteric artery, a visceral branch of the abdominal aorta at the level of 1st lumber vertebra running within the root of mesentery. These arteries branch anastomose with each other to form a series orders of arterial arches. The last order of arterial arch gives off straight arteries to each side wall of the small intestine.

The veins of small intestine accompany with the corresponding arteries and unite to form the superior mesenteric vein, which lies right side of artery. It goes upward behind the neck of pancreas and unites with the splenic vein, the hepatic portal vein.

The lymphatic drainage of the jejunum and ileum goes to the mesenteric lymph nodes placed along the branches of the superior mesenteric artery, then they converges to the superior mesenteric lymph nodes.

The nerve supply is the autonomic nerves.

4.2　The anatomy of vermiform appendix

4.2.1　Position

It lies in the right inguinal region. The root of it attaches to the posteriomedial wall of cecum, 2~3 cm below the ileocecal valve, where is an union of 3 colic bands. The apex is variable: preileal position (28%), pelvic (26%), retrocecal (24%), retroileal (8%) and subcecal (6%). The root of it is constant, the surface projection is:

McBurney point corresponds to the attachment of the appendix to the cecum, it lies at the junction of the middle and lateral thirds of a line drawn from the umbilicus to the right anterior superior iliac spine.

Lanz point is a junction of the right and middle thirds of a line between both sides of anterior superior iliac spine.

4.2.2　Mesoappendix

The mesoappendix is a triangular peritoneal fold which continuous with lower part of mesentery, appendicular vessels lie in its free border.

4.2.3　Blood supply

Appendicular artery comes from the ileocolic artery, enters the mesoappendix and goes along the free margin.

Appendicular veins enter into the ileocolic vein, and then the superior mesenteric vein, hepatic portal vein.

4.3 The anatomy of the colon

4.3.1 Position and relations

The colon starts from the upper part of cecum and terminate in the superior part of rectum, it surrounds the jejunum and ileum. There are 4 parts: ascending, transverse, descending and sigmoid colons.

Ascending colon is an interperitoneal organ which is about 15 cm in length. It is continuous with the cecum at the level of ileocecal junction inferiorly and extends upward to the right lobe of liver, continuous with transverse colon by the right colic flexure (hepatic flexure). It's related to right colic sulcus lateral side, right mesenteric sinus and ileum, duodenum medial side, right lobe of liver and gallbladder superiorly and anteriorly.

Transverse colon is intraperitoneal organ, which is about 50 cm long. It starts from right colic flexure and runs to left side to the spleen continuous with descending colon by the left colic flexure (splenic flexure).

Descending colon is about 20 cm long and interperitomeal organ. It starts from the left colic flexure in the left hypochondriac region and runs downward continues to sigmoid colon distally.

Sigmoid colon is about 45 cm in length, but has a greater variation. It continuous with descending colon at the level of iliac crest and with rectum at level of 3rd sacral vertebra. Sigmoid mesocolon suspends and fixes it to the pelvic wall.

4.3.2 Blood supply, lymphatic drainage and innervation

The right (or ascending) and middle colic arteries come from superior mesenteric artery, the left (or descending) and sigmoid arteries from inferior mesenteric artery. The colic arteries and the terminal branch of ileocecal anastomoses with each other to form an arterial arch in the medial border of colon, it is called colic marginal artery which gives off longer and shorter branches to enter the wall of colon. The veins of colon drain into superior and inferior mesenteric veins respectively, and then into the portal vein.

Lymphatic drainage and nerves please refer textbook for details.

4.4 Hepatic portal vein

The hepatic portal vein is a shorter and thicker venous trunk, which is about 6~8 cm long and 1~1.2 cm in diameter. It drains venous blood from single viscera of abdominal and pelvic cavities(except the lower part of rectum, anal canal and liver) into liver.

4.4.1 Formation

The hepatic portal vein is usually formed by the union of the superior mesenteric vein and splenic vein behind the neck of pancreas. Ablut the type of hepatic portal vein, please refer the textbook for details.

4.4.2 Relations

The hepatic portal vein runs upward to the hilum of liver behind the pancreas, superior part of duodenum and inside of the hepatoduodenal ligament. The inferior vena cava is behind it, the common bile duct is right and anterior, the proper hepatic artery is left and anterior.

4.4.3　Tributaries

The main tributaries of hepatic portal vein include the superior mesenteric vein, inferior mesenteric vein, splenic vein, left gastric vein, right gastric vein, cystic vein and paraumbilical vein.

4.4.4　Communications between the hepatic portal vein and systemic vein

There are several collateral anastomoses between them, such as from the esophageal venous plexus, rectal venous plexus, paraumbilical venous rete and the Retzius veins (small anastomotic veins between abdominal viscera and tributaries of inferior vena cava). These anastomoses are confined in normal. The collateral circulations occurs in portal hypertension, please refer the textbook for details.

5　The retroperitoneal space

The retroperitoneal space is between the parietal peritoneum and endoabdominal fascia of posterior abdominal wall, extending from diaphragm downward to the sacral promontory and pelvic inlet. Many important structures, such as the kidney, ureter, adrenal gland, abdominal aorta, inferior vena cava, sympathetic trunk, are in it.

5.1　The anatomy of kidney

5.1.1　Position

The kidney is located on both sides of the lumbar segment of the spinal column. Due to the location of liver, the right kidney is 1~2 cm lower than the left kidney.

Right kidney—the superior border of T12~L3 vertebrae, 12th rib across back of upper part of it.

Left kidney—the lower border of T11~L2 vertebrae, 12th rib across back of middle part of it.

In the posterior abdominal wall, the angle formed by lateral edge of the erector spinae with 12th rib, is called renal angle.

5.1.2　Relations

The kidney is related to the adrenal gland superiorly.

Medially the left kidney is related to the abdominal aorta, the right kidney to inferior vena cava, the inner rear respectively related to the sympathetic trunk.

Left kidney is adjacent to the stomach, pancreas, jejunum and the left colic flexure; right kidney is adjacent to the right lobe of the liver, right colic flexure and the descending part of duodenum anteriorly respectively.

Behind the 12th rib, there are diaphragm and the pleural cavity; the subcostal, iliohypogastric and ilioinguinal nerves in front of the psoas major and quadratus lumborum from up down.

5.1.3 Renal hilum and renal pedicle

The central depression in the medial border of kidney is called the renal hilum, renal pelvis, blood and lymphatic vessels, and nerves within the renal pedicle, which enter or leave the kidney.

The arrangement of main structures, from front to back is: the renal vein, the renal artery and the renal pelvis; from up to down is: renal artery, renal vein and renal pelvis.

5.1.4 Renal artery and renal segments

The renal artery comes from side of the abdominal aorta at the level of 1st lumbar vertebral body, it is divided into anterior and posterior branches. In the renal sinus, the anterior one divides into superior, superioanterior, inferioanterior and inferior segmental arteries. Each artery was distributed in the corresponding region of the renal parenchyma, i. e., the segment of the kidney. There were five renal segments: the superior segment, the superioranterior segment, the inferioanterior segment, the inferior segment and the posterior segment.

The accessory renal artery should be taken care during the operation of kidney.

The renal veins enter to the inferior vena cava.

5.1.5 Coverings

From outside in, there are the renal fascia, adipose capsule and fibrous capsule in turn. The renal fascia and adipose fascia play a role of fixation for kidney.

5.2 The anatomy of suprarenal gland

5.2.1 Position

It locates on both sides of the vertebral column, which is equivalent to the height of the 11th thoracic vertebrae, just above the kidney. The left suprarenal gland is semilunar shape, right one is triangular.

5.2.2 Relations

In front of the left adrenal gland, there are stomach, pancreas and splenic artery, the medial side is the abdominal aorta, the back is the diaphragm. In front of the right adrenal gland is the liver, the medial is inferior vena cava.

5.2.3 Blood supply

The arteries can be divided into superior, middle and inferior suprarenal arteries, which were derived from the inferior phrenic, abdominal aorta and renal artery. The adrenal vein usually has 1 branch in each side. The left suprarenal vein drains to the left renal vein, and the right one to the inferior vena cava directly.

5.3 Abdominal ureter

The ureter is located lateral to the spine, from lower end of the renal pelvis to urinary bladder, a total length of about 25~30 cm. There are 3 parts: the abdominal, pelvic and the intramural parts; 3 physiological structures: the ureteropelvic junction, inlet of pelvis and the intramural part. The abdominal ureter is about 13~14 cm long, which body surface projection is equal to the semilunar line of the anterior abdominal wall.

The relations of both ureters are different. Anterior to the upper part of the right ureter are the descending part of duodenum, right colic and ileocolic arteries, root of the mesentery and right testicular(or ovarian) vessels; in front of lower part are the ileocecum and vermiform appendix. In front of the left one are duodenojejunal flexure, left colic artery, left testicular (ovarian) vessels, and the sigmoid mesocolon.

5.4 Abdominal aorta

5.4.1   Position and relations

The abdominal aorta is continuous with the thoracic aorta at the level of 12th thoracic vertebra(the aortic hiatus of the diaphragm), then it runs downward in front of spine to the 4th lumbar vertebral body and bifurcates into right and left common iliac arteries.

5.4.2   Branches

▶ Parietal branches

There are the inferior phrenic artery (1 pair), lumbar arteries(4 pairs), and the median sacral artery(single).

▶ Visceral branches

Single branches including the celiac trunk, superior mesenteric artery, and the inferior mesenteric artery

Paired branches including the middle suprarenal artery, renal artery, and the testicular (or ovarian) artery.

5.5 Inferior vena cava

5.5.1   Position and relations

The inferior vena cava is formed by the right and left common iliac veins at the level of 5th lumbar vertebra. It goes upward right and anterior to the spine to the opening of vena cava of diaphragm at the level of 8th thoracic vertebra.

5.5.2   Tributaries

There are the common iliac veins, lumbar veins, renal veins, inferior phrenic veins, hepatic veins, the left suprarenal vein and left testicular(or ovarian) vein.

5.6 Lumbar sympathetic trunk

The paired lumbar sympathetic trunks lie on the sides of the vertebrral bodies. Each is continuous to the thoracic sympathetic trunk superiorly and pelvic part inferiorly. The left trunk lies to the left side of the abdominal aorta but slightly behind; the right one lies behind the inferior vena cava.

Section 2

Dissection and observation

Ⅰ. Abdominal wall

1　Position and incisions

Set the body in supine position, make incisions as following instructions.

● From the xiphoid process of sternum cut downward along the midline, make a circular incision in the umbilicus to the pubic symphysis.

● From the level of the xiphoid cut a way to anterior axillary line.

● From the pubic symphysis to the anterior superior iliac spine.

The incisions should be superficial in case of damaging the structures.

2　Procedures

2.1　Dissect superficial structures

2.1.1　Identify the Camper's and the Scarpa's fascia

Cut the superficial fascia gently along the midline, distinguish the fat(Camper') and membranous(Scarpa') layer below the level of the umbilicus. Open the membranous layer transversely along the line between the anterior superior iliac spine and the umbilicus, inserting a handle or a finger, adhesion can seen in the midline with the linea alba. Below the inguinal ligament about 1.5 cm, it is the fascia lata; in the pubic tubercle, it across the front of the pubis and continuous with the dartos coat and Colles' fascia.

2.1.2　Cutaneous nerves and superficial vessels

The anterior and the lateral cutaneous branches of lower six pairs of intercostal nerves emerging out on both sides of the midline and in the midaxillary line, distributed in the abdominal wall.

The iliohypogastric and the ilioinguinal nerves are situated under muscles which passes medially and downward, they distribute to the skin.

Try to recognize the superficial epigastric artery, the superficial circumflex iliac artery and accompanying veins.

2. 2   Dissect deep structures

2.2.1   Rectus abdominis and its sheath

Observe the semilunar line on the lateral border of rectus sheath, open the anterior sheath vertically at its midline, turn to the sides, and separate the tendinous intersections (3~4) connected the anterior sheath to the rectus. Then lift the lateral border of the rectus muscles, identify the branches of lower intercostal nerves and subcostal nerve through the posterior rectus sheath into the sheath. Cut off the rectus abdominis in midpoint, turn it up and down; observe the posterior rectus sheath, the lower edge of it goes below the umbilical 4~5 cm, the arcuate line. Find the superior and inferior epigastric vessels.

2.2.2   Linea alba

Carefully observe the anatomic features of the linea alba, it is at the midline between the rectus sheath both sides.

2.2.3   Muscles

Observe the range of external oblique muscle, fibers direction and the three structures formed by the aponeurosis.

The inguinal ligament is attached to the anterior superior iliac spine and the pubic tubercle.

The subcutaneous (superficial) inguinal ring is located lateral and above the pubic tubercle.

The lacunar ligament is medial part fibers of the inguinal ligament and turns back to the pectineal ligament.

Cut the externus obliquus abdominis from the anterior superior iliac spine to the 12th rib along the midaxillary line, then cut the muscle along the costal arch and the anterior superior iliac spine to the semilunar line respectively; cut the internus obliquus abdominis and the transversus abdominis same as the externus. Separate the muscles bluntly by a finger, reflect muscle flaps medially layer by layer. Be careful not to incise too deeply, avoid injuring the deep muscles and intercostal nerves between muscles.

2.2.4   Inguinal canal

Cut the aponeurosis of externus obliquus abdominis along semilunar line down to the pubic tubercle. Lift and reflect aponeurosis laterally and downward carefully, pay attention to the medial and lateral crura of superficial ring of inguinal canal, the external spermatic fascia, the cremaster, genital branch of the iliohypogastric nerve, ilioinguinal nerve and genitofemoral nerve. Protect the nerves, cut off the internal oblique muscle from inguinal ligament, turn it medially. Lift the spermatic cord and observe from the superficial ring of inguinal canal to deep (abdominal) ring. Abdominal ring is 1.5~2 cm above the midpoint of the inguinal ligament, a bag-shaped downward of transverse fascia continuation with the internal spermatic fascia. Look for the inferior epigastric artery lateral to the deep ring. The structures will be observed adjacent to the spermatic cord, formed the walls of inguinal canal.

II. Peritoneum and peritoneal cavity

1 Open the anterior abdominal wall

Turn back the anterior thoracic wall, cut the remaining lower ribs, and then continue to cut down the abdominal wall to anterior superior iliac spine.

Cut the attachment of the diaphragm to the sternum in point of xiphoid process, and then to both sides of ribs attachment.

The anterior thoracoabdominal wall is opened downward, cut off the attachment to the anterior abdominal wall of the falciform ligament of liver and round ligament of liver.

2 Exploration of peritoneum and peritoneal cavity

The naked eye and hand touch can be used for exploration. Examine the positions and sizes of the abdominal organs and investigate them with the regions of the abdomen (the four regions or the nine regions) without damaging the peritoneum and the structures covered by the peritoneum.

2.1 Exploration of the supracolic compartment

2.1.1 Observation of the liver

Lift the diaphragm in the right hypochondriac region, observe the falciform ligament, coronary ligament and triangular ligament above the liver. Lift up the liver, observe the gallbladder, the fundus of the gallbladder extends beyond the anterior margin of the liver usually.

Observe the lesser omentum when the liver is lifted up and the stomach is pulled down. The left part of it is the hepatogastric ligament, and the right part of it is the hepatoduodinal ligament. Omental foramen is behind the right free margin of lesser omentum. Below the right lobe of the liver, the right kidney can be touched.

2.1.2 Observation of the stomach

Observe the adjacent organs in front of the stomach.

Touch the fundus of the stomach below the left half of the diaphragm. The cardia and the esophagus can be touched along the fundus of the stomach to the right; along the lesser curvature of the stomach to right the pylorus can be touched. The greater curvature of the stomach is attached by the greater omentum.

2.1.3　Observation of the spleen

In the left hypochondriac, left side of stomach, try to find the spleen. Observe the ligaments of the spleen, such as the splenogastric, the splenocolic and the splenorenal ligaments. The left kidney can be felt from the right side of the spleorenal ligament.

2.2　Exploration of the infracolic compartment

The greater omentum is turned upward, the large and small intestine can be seen. The jejunum and ileum was surrounded by the "?" shaped large intestine, how to distinguish the large and small intestine?

To determine the initial part of jejunum, the greater omentum and the transverse colon, the transverse mesocolon can be turned up. Touch the spine in the root of transverse mesocolon, and slide to the left side, you can touch the duodenal suspensory ligament, the origin of the jejunum, the duodenojejunal flexure connected to it.

Observation of the root of mesentery: turn the whole small intestine to the right side, observe the attachment and length of the root. Lift the intestine and mesentery up, and observe the blood vessels in it.

The cecum lies in the right iliac fossa, and the vermiform appendix may be found along the colic bands in front of it. Observe the position of the appendix and the mesoappendix.

Observe the position of the ascending colon, right colic flexure, transverse colon, left colic flexure, descending colon and sigmoid colon.

2.3　Exploration of pelvic cavity

The positions of rectum, urinary bladder, the prostate, the seminal vesicals and the ampulla of the ductus deferens, the vesicorectal pouch should be observed in the male pelvic cavity.

Observe the position of the uterus, uterine tube, ovary, rectum and urinary bladder, the broad and the round ligaments of the uterus, the proper and the suspensory ligaments of the ovary; the uterovesical pouch and the uterorectal pouch.

Ⅲ. Supracolic compartment

Lifting up the liver while pushing down the stomach, the anterior layer of lesser omentum can be cut along the lesser curvature of the stomach. Look for the left gastric artery and vein near the cardia, find out the esophageal branch from the artery, and pay attention to the accessory hepatic artery from it. Lymph nodes arrange along the blood vessels should be observed.

Opening the peritoneum in front of the abdominal part of esophagus, the anterior trunk of vagus nerve can be find. Pay attention to the relationship between the vagus nerves and left gastric vessels.

Trace the arterial arch along the lesser curvature of stomach to right, clean out the right gastric artery, and then the proper hepatic artery.

The structures of the hepatoduodenal ligament.

The anterior layer of the hepatoduodenal ligament is opened longitudinally, proper hepatic artery is on the left, up to the hepatic hilum, which is divided into left and right branches.

From the posterior wall of the right hepatic artery, the cystic artery was found to the neck of gallbladder behind hepatic duct. Pay attention to the variation of cystic artery.

Dissect the common bile duct in the right of proper hepatic artery, clean out the cystic duct and proper hepatic duct upward, and down to the medial wall of the descending duodenum.

Look for the hepatic portal vein behind the common bile duct and the proper hepatic artery, and then trace up to the hepatic hilum, down to the superior edge of the head of pancreas.

Trace the left gastric artery to the celiac artery when the lesser curvature of the stomach is pushed downward gently. The celiac lymph nodes and the celiac plexus surrounding the celiac artery can be observed and cleaned out to expose the celiac artery.

Clean up the three branches of the celiac artery, on the left up to the left gastric artery, right to the common hepatic artery and left down to the splenic artery.

Open the greater omentum along the greater curvature, dissect right gastroepiploic artery out to the right, and then trace to the gastroduodenal artery below the pylorus; dissect the left gastroepiploic artery to the left, then to the hilum of spleen. Observe the anastomosis position of left and right gastroepiploic arteries, and observe the branches to the stomach and the infrapyloric lymph nodes.

To expose the pancreas, cut the greater omentum transversely below the left and right gastroepiploic arteries, and then pull up the stomach. Transect the peritoneum in the superior border of pancreas to find the splenic artery bended left side to the hilum of spleen and the pancreatic branches of splenic artery. Clear the short gastric artery and the splenic branches of the splenic artery near the hilum of spleen. Pull forward the upper edge of the pancreas find the splenic vein below the splenic artery, the hepatic portal vein, tracing right side.

Turn the greater curvature of the stomach upward, look for the origin of the posterior gastric artery in the middle of the splenic artery behind the peritoneum of posterior wall of omental bursa. It goes to left and upward, then into the gastrophrenic ligament to the posterior wall of fundus of the stomach near the cardia finally. Posterior gastric vein goes with artery.

After the stomach is turned right upward, look for the posterior trunk of the vagus nerve out behind the abdominal part of esophagus.

Find the gastroduodenal artery behind pylorus of stomach, trace up to the beginning, clean out the superior pancreaticoduodenal artery and the right gastroepiploic artery down.

Ⅳ. Infracolic compartment

To expose the root of the mesentery, the greater omentum, transverse colon and its mesocolon are turned upward. The jejunum and ileum all are pushed to the lower left, the mesentery is tension. The root of the mesentery was opened longitudinally in anterior layer, clean out the superior mesenteric artery and the vein of namesake on right. To observe the mesenteric lymph nodes and the nerve plexus along the vessels.

Dissect the jejunal and ileal arteries from the left edge of the superior mesenteric artery. These arteries in the mesentery branch out and anastomosize each other and form the arterial arches increased from the top down gradually, about 1~4 levels. A straight artery from the convex of arch enter into the wall of intestine.

At the right edge of the superior mesenteric artery, from inferior to superior the ileocolic artery, right colic artery and middle colic artery are dissected in turn. At the beginning of the superior mesenteric artery, try to find the inferior pancreaticoduodenal artery. Dissect the appendical artery in the free margin of the mesoappendix, up to its origin.

Pushing all the jejunum and ileum right side, the peritoneum is opened at the center of the lower abdomen, to find out the origin of the inferior mesenteric artery above the bifurcation of abdominal aorta about 4 cm, and then clean up the branches from up to down in turn: the left colic artery, the sigmoid arteries and the superior rectal artery. Observe the inferior mesenteric vein, which is located on the left side of the same artery.

Observe the colic marginal artery in inner edge of the colon, it is arterial anastomosis of colic arteries and paralleled with colon. There are long and short terminal arteries from the marginal artery to the colic wall directly and vertically.

Observe and trace the superior and inferior mesenteric veins upward to the posterior of the neck of the pancreas joining with the splenic vein, the hepatic portal vein.

Ⅴ. Retroperitoneal space

1 Abdominal aorta and its branches

The remainder parietal peritoneum of posterior abdominal wall was removed to expose the retroperitoneal space. Remove the lymph nodes around the abdominal aorta and inferior vena cava after observing, clean out the root of celiac, superior mesenteric and inferior mesenteric arteries carefully, observe the celiac ganglia, celiac plexus, superior mesenteric plexus, inferior mesenteric plexus and abdominal aortic plexus. Trace and clean up the branches of the abdominal aorta as follow.

▶ Renal artery

Below the superior mesenteric artery, the renal arteries originate from the abdominal aorta at right. The right side is longer and slightly lower than the left side. The renal artery has a branch to the adrenal gland, which is called the inferior suprarenal artery. Pay attention to whether the existence of the accessory renal artery, from the renal artery or abdominal aorta to the upper or lower ends of the kidney without passing renal hilum.

▶ Middle suprarenal artery

It originates from the lateral wall of the abdominal aorta at roughly the same level, with the superior mesenteric artery, then goes up and laterally to the suprarenal gland.

▶ Testicular (ovarian) artery

The testicular artery comes from the anterior wall of the abdominal aorta about 2nd lumbar height slightly below renal artery, goes down along the front of psoas major, to the height of the lower edge of the 4th lumbar, crosses in front of the ureter and iliac vessels obliquely to the deep inguinal ring.

The origin and course of ovarian artery in the abdomen is similar to that of testicular artery. Trace it to the suspensory ligament of the ovary.

▶ Inferior phrenic artery

It comes from the abdominal aorta just a little lower to the aortic hiatus of the diaphragm. The left inferior phrenic artery passes behind the esophagus, and the right one behind the inferior vena cava. The superior suprarenal artery originates from the origin of it, and distribute to the suprarenal gland.

▶ Lumbar artery

There are 4 pairs coming from the posterior wall of the abdominal aorta at the level of upper 4 lumbar vertebrae, and go laterally behind the quadratus lumborum to distribute in the posterior abdominal wall.

▶ Median sacral artery

As a single, originates from the posterior wall at the bifurcation of the abdominal aorta, goes down in front of the spine.

2　Inferior vena cava

Observe the veins accompanying the paired visceral branches and parietal branches of the abdominal aorta, their relation with the inferior vena cava.

3　Kidney and suprarenal gland

Open the peritoneum in front of the kidney longitudinally, observe the renal fascia, adipose capsule and fibrous capsule.

Clean out and observe the renal vein, the renal artery and the renal pelvis in the renal pedicle and renal hilum.

Dissect the left suprarenal gland in the upper pole of the left kidney, the right one is not easy to dissect because the liver.

4   Ureter

Find out the ureter on both sides of the lumbar spine by removing the parietal peritoneum, and then trace and clean up to the renal pelvis, down to the pelvic cavity. In the abdomen, the testicular or the ovarian vessels pass through the ureter posteriorly, and at the entrance of the pelvis, the iliac blood vessels pass through the ureter in front.

Review of the course, the stenosis and the decussation with the vessels of the ureter.

5   Sympathetic trunk

On the left side of the abdominal aorta, the left lumbar sympathetic trunk was found along the medial margin of the psoas major. Look for the right lumbar sympathetic trunk behind the inferior vena cava, observe the lumbar sympathetic ganglia and the communicating branches.

Section 3

Clinical application

I. Anatomical basis of the hernias

There are inguinal hernias and femoral hernia in the inguinal region. The inguinal hernias can be divided into the direct and indirect(oblique) hernias. In direct hernia, the viscera protrude forward to the inguinal triangle, medial to inferior epigastric vessels, emerge from the superficial inguinal ring. In indirect hernia, however, the viscera enter the deep inguinal ring, lateral to the inferior epigastric vessels, traverse the inguinal canal emerge from same site with the direct one. So the neck of hernial sac of the inguinal hernias are above the inguinal ligament.

In the femoral hernia, the abdominal contents protrude downward from the femoral ring of the femoral canal in the femoral triangle, therefore the neck of hernial sac of femoral hernia is just below the inguinal ligament.

II. Clinical relevance of the peritoneum

The peritoneum is a smooth, glistening and serous membranous that lines the abdominopelvic wall and surface of the viscera. The parietal and visceral layers continue to each other and form the peritoneal cavity. It is complete closed in male, while it communicates with the outside through the uterine tube, uterus and vagina in female.

The peritoneum, especially the parietal layer, has absorption power. Abdominal or pelvic surgical patients should be in Fowler's position, so inflammatory effusion would gravitate down into the pelvis. The peritoneum in the subphrenic region has greater absorptive capacity due to a larger surface.

The peritoneum provides a smooth surface that permits free movement of abdominopelvic organs. The greater omentum, a remarkable structure formed by peritoneum, is rich in vessels, lymphatics and fatty tissue, contains numerous fixed macrophages which perform an important protective function and can limit the spreading of infection in the peritoneal cavity.

. Clinical relevance of the stomac

The lower part of anterior wall of stomach is related to the anterior abdominal wall directly, so we can palpate the stomach below the substernal angle. The posterior wall of stomach is related to pancreas closely by the omental bursa, therefore the ulcer or the cancer of stomach may invade the pancreas and adhere to it, and the infection may lead to an abscess in the omental bursa after operation on its posterior wall.

The parasympathetic nerve supplying the stomach is the vagus nerve, it is to control the secretion of acid and contraction of stomach wall. Excess acid secretion may cause ulcer in the stomach or the duodenum. So a high selective vagatomy is done during which only the gastric branches of anterior and posterior vagus trunk are sectioned far from the pylorus, has a desired effect on the secretion of acid without the contraction of the stomach.

IV. Gallbladder

It locates in the fossa for gallbladder on the inferior surface of liver, and it attaches to liver by loose connective tissue in which there are small vessels and even small bile channel. In hence, the ligation should be done not only the cystic vessels and cystic duct but the small tubules in order to avoid bleeding and leakage of the bile during the cholecystectomy.

V. Ileocecal region

The terminal part of ileum, cecum and vermiform appendix form an important surgical unit, called ileocecal region, in clinic. The end of ileum enters the cecum posteromedially at a right angle usually, the ileocecal intussusception may occur, especially in children, because the diameter of the cecum is about three times larger than that of ileum.

The Meckel's diverticulum is one of the most common malformation of the ileum. It is a finger-like blind pouch, 2~5 cm long, projecting from the antimesenteric border. When it becomes inflamed and perforated, it results in symptoms similar to those of appendicitis.

The vermiform appendix is s hook-like, spiral in shape. In adult, it has thicker wall, smaller lumen, and narrower orifice than that in children. The appendicitis in adult is obstructive usually and perforative, rarely in children, so the appendicectomy should be performed as early as possible. The symptoms of appendicitis are associated to the different positions of apex of appendix, the root of it is fixed.

VI. Kidney

The kidney lies in the retroperitoneal space on both sides of spine at the level T11~L3 vertebrae. It may be located in lower abdomen, pelvic cavity, and even both on same side abnormally.

The variations of renal vessels are common, the accessory renal artery occurs in 42% of individuals. The upper (lower) polar artery arises from the abdominal aorta or renal artery, enters the upper (lower) segment of kidney doesn't passing through the hilum of kidney. Attention must be paid while diagnosis and operation.

Section 4

Ask yourself

1. Why inguinal area is the predilection site for hernia? How to distinguish the inguinal hernia from femoral hernia? And how to distinguish direct inguinal hernia from indirect inguinal hernia?

2. Which peripheral organ may be adherence to when ulcer of posterior gastric perforation happened?

3. A patient diagnosed with perforating appendicitis stays consecutive high body temperature after appendicitis. There are three possible diagnosis: the subdiaphragmatic abscess, subhepatic abscess or pelvic abscess. Try to explain the situation with your anatomy knowledge.

4. What disease of adjacent organs should be identified with appendicitis? How to find the appendix during the appendectomy?

5. Try to explain the four major symptoms of pancreatic head carcinoma, such as the enlargement of duodenal ring (or duodenal obstruction), obstructive jaundice, ascites and edema of the lower extremities by anatomy.

6. A female patient in her forties is hospitalized for cholelithiasis, the doctor decided to perform cholecystectomy and laparoscopic common bile duct exploration after physical examination. Try to answer the following questions.

ⅰ. Which parts can the extrahepatic biliary duct be divided? Where is the opening at last?

ⅱ. Which is the easiest way to find the cystic artery for ligation in cholecystectomy?

ⅲ. How to find the common bile duct during the operation?

ⅳ. Which parts can the common bile duct be divided? What important adjacent structures is related to each parts?

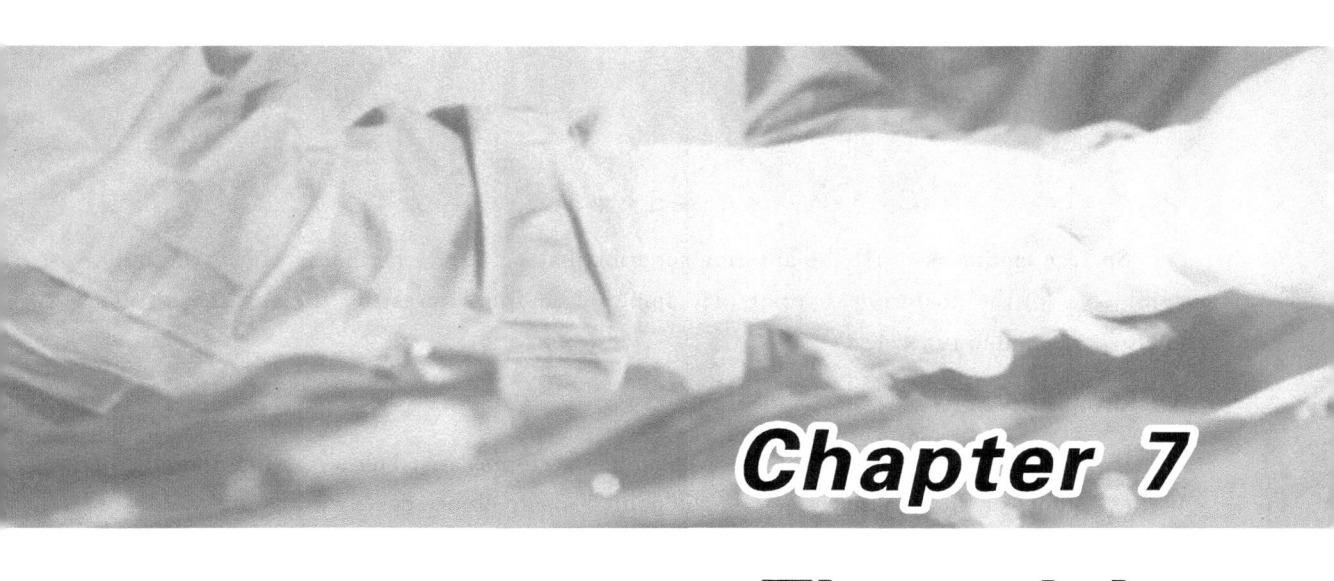

Chapter 7

The pelvis

Section 1

Review

Surface landmark: ① the anterior superior iliac spine ② the iliac crest ③ the pubic symphysis ④ the posterior superior iliac spine ⑤ the pubic crest ⑥ the tubercle of iliac crest ⑦ the pubic tubercle.

1 Rhomboid area

Touch the spinous process of the 5th lumbar vertebra, just below the line joining the highest points of the two iliac crests at the point 1.5 cm. Trace downward along the posterior median line to get the tip of the coccyx which located 5 cm posterosuperior to the anus. Join the posterior superior iliac spines with the 5th lumbar spinous process and the tip of the coccyx respectively to demarcate the rhomboid area of the lumbosacral region.

2 Sacral hiatus

Make a line connecting the upper and lower angles of the rhomboid area, palpate the median sacral crest which is formed by the fusion of the sacral spinous processes. Lateral to this crest, find the intermediate sacral, the lower end of this crest is very prominent, known as crest cornu which is formed by the lower articular process of the 5th sacral vertebral. Between the sacral cornu of both sides and lower end of the median sacral crest palpate as fossa, deep to the fossa, it is the sacral hiatus. In clinical medicine, the sacral anesthesia is done by injecting the anesthetic into the sacral canal by way of this hiatus.

Ⅱ. Boundaries and divisions

The pelvis contains the hip bones, the sacrum, the coccyx and dense ligaments that bound them. The pelvic is divided into the greater and lesser pelvis. The pelvic wall includes bones, joints and ligaments lines by muscles which are wrapped by fascia.

The lateral boundaries of the perineum are the inferior rami of the pubes, the rami of ischia and the sacrotuberous ligaments. The perineum has a large posterior anal region and a small anterior urogenital region by a line joining the anterior parts of the ischial tuberosities.

Ⅲ. Main contents

1 Pelvic walls and pelvic diaphragm

1.1 Pelvic walls

▶ Bony pelvis

It includes two hip bones, the sacrum and coccyx. They are connected by two sacroiliac—the pubic symphysis and the sacrococcygeal joint.

The pelvis has two parts which are separated by the oblique plane of the superior aperture of the lesser pelvis, this plane runs from the promontory of sacrum to the upper border of the public symphysis. The greater pelvis is formed by iliac fossa and a part of the abdominal wall. The part posteroinferior to this plane is the lesser pelvis. The cavity of the lesser pelvis is C-shaped with a long curved posterosuperior wall formed by the sacrum and coccyx, the lateral wall is formed by the ilium, body of the pubis, ischium, sacrotuberous and sacrospinous ligaments. These two ligaments and the greater and lesser ischial notches form the greater and lesser sciatic foramina, through which blood vessels, nerves, muscles, and tendons pass to the gluteal region and perineum.

▶ Muscles of the pelvic walls

Including obturator internus and piriformis.

1.2 Pelvic diaphragm

The muscles of pelvic diaphragm comprises levator ani and coccygeus. The superior and inferior fasciae of pelvic diaphragm cover the superior and inferior surfaces of the muscles. The pelvic diaphragm separates the pelvis from the perineum.

2 Pelvic fascia

It can be divided into the parietal pelvic fascia, visceral pelvic fascia and fascia of pelvic diaphragm.

● Parietal pelvic fascia It covers the anterior, posterior and lateral walls of the pelvis as well as the obturator internus and piriformis.

● Visceral pelvic fascia It covers the organs, blood vessels and nerves in the pelvis.

● Fascia of pelvic diaphragm It lines the floor of the pelvis, named the superior and inferior fascia of pelvic diaphragm.

● Fascial spaces Please refer the textbook.

3 Blood vessels, lymphatic drainage and nerves of the pelvis

3.1 The common iliac vessels and lymph nodes

The abdominal aorta divides into the right and left common iliac arteries in front of the 4th lumbar vertebra. The common iliac artery runs along the medial border of the psoas major muscle to the front of the sacroiliac joint, where it ends by bifurcating into the external and internal iliac arteries. Behind the common iliac artery lies the common iliac vein.

3.2 The external iliac vessels and lymph nodes

The external iliac artery passes downward along the medial border at first and then the front of psoas muscle to the back of the inguinal ligament at the mid-inguinal point, where its name changes to femoral artery. The external iliac vein lies medial to the external iliac artery. Along the sides of the external iliac artery, there are several lymph nodes, named external iliac lymph nodes, the efferent vessels of which are drained into the common iliac nodes.

3.3 The internal iliac vessels and lymph nodes

The internal iliac artery is about 4 cm long and runs downward into the lesser pelvis, passing in the pelvic fascia posterolaterally, to end by dividing into anterior and posterior trunks. The internal iliac vein accompanies the artery on its medial side.

▶ The branches of the anterior trunk

The parietal branches are the obturator artery and the inferior gluteal artery. The obturator artery runs anteroinferiorly along side wall of the pelvis to the obturator canal. It is accompanied by its respective nerve and vein. The visceral branches of the anterior trunk are:

- Unbilical artery
- Inferior vesical artery
- Inferior rectal artery
- Uterine artery
- Internal pudendal artery
- Branches of the posterior trunk

3.4 Other arteries in the pelvis

- Superior rectal artery
- Ovarian artery
- Median sacral artery

3.5 Pelvic venous plexuses

- Rectal venous plexuses
- Vesical venous plexuses

- Uterovaginal venous plexuses
- Pudendal venous plexuses

3.6　Nerves of the pelvis

- Sacral plexus
- Pelvic sympathetic trunks
- Pelvic splanchnic nerve
- Superior and inferior hypogastric plexus
- Obturator nerve

4　Viscera in the pelvic cavity

4.1　The relationship between the viscera and peritoneum in the pelvic cavity

The urinary bladder has four surfaces in the male. The superior surface and upper portion of the fundus are covered by peritoneum, the fundus of bladder is in close relation with the ampulla ductus deferentis and seminal vesicle. At the base of the broad ligament of uterus, the anterior and posterior layers are continuous with peritoneum of the vesicouterine pouch and rectouterine pouch respectively.

4.2　Urinary bladder

4.2.1　Position, shape and relations

The urinary bladder rests against the pubis. When it is empty, it lies entirely in the lesser pelvis; once it is filling, it may raise beyond the superior border of pubic symphysis. The empty bladder has the shape of a pyramid with its apex situated anteriorly and its triangular fundus posteroinferiorly. Between the apex and the fundus is the body of bladder.

4.2.2　Interior feature

The trigone of bladder is on the interior of the fundus of bladder. The two ureteric orifices form two lateral angles and the internal urethral orifice forms its lower angle.

4.2.3　Blood supply, lymphatic drainage and innervation

- Superior vesical artery
- Inferior vesical artery
- Veins
- Lymphatic drainage
- Nerves

4.3　Rectum

The rectum lies in front of the sacrum and coccyx. It begins at the pelvic surface of the 3rd sacral vertebra as the continuation of the sigmoid colon. The part of the rectum superior to the pelvic diaphragm is the pelvic part and below this diaphragm is the anal canal.

4.3.1 Interior features

There are 6~10 longitudinal folds called the anal columns, whose lower ends are united by semilunar folds, the anal valves. The small pockets formed by the lower ends of the anal columns and anal valves are the anal sinuses. The lower ends of anal columns and the bases of the anal valves form a circular dentate line.

4.3.2 Relations

In the male, it is separated from the fundus of bladder, seminal vesicle, ampulla ductus deferentis by the rectovesical pouch; below the pouch it is in relation with the fundus of bladder, seminal vesicle, ampulla ductus deferentis, prostate and the ureter. In the female, it is anteriorly separated from uterus and posterior part of fornix of vagina by the rectouterine pouch; below this pouch, it is separated from the vagina by fascial septum.

4.3.3 Blood supply, lymphatic drainage and nerves of the rectum

▶ Arteries

The superior rectal artery is the continuation of the inferior mesenteric artery. It descends in the sigmoid mesocolon to the beginning of rectum, where it divides into right and left branches, entering the lateral wall of rectum. The inferior rectal artery is a branch of internal iliac artery supplying the lower part of the rectum. The anal artery is a branch of internal pudendal artery supplying the part of anal canal below the dentate line.

▶ Veins

The internal rectal venous plexus is the submucous in the upper part of the rectum and subcutaneous in the anal canal. It can be divided into superior and inferior parts by the dentate line.

▶ Lymphatic drainage

The lymphatic vessels of the rectum drain into the inferior mesenteric lymph nodes, internal iliac lymph nodes and the superficial inguinal lymph nodes.

▶ Nerves

The part above the dentate line is supplied by sympathetic and parasympathetic nerves. The latter is the main nerve to regulate the function of the rectum. It comes from the pelvic splanchnic nerve and passes through the pelvic plexus.

4.4 Pelvic part of the ureter

The ureter enters the pelvis at the bifurcation of the common iliac artery and descends immediately in front of the internal iliac artery.

4.5 Prostate

Its size is about the size of a walnut, but is, in general, cone-shaped with its base against the neck of bladder. The apex of the cone rests on the urogenital diaphragm. The part between the apex and base is the body which has anterior, inferolateral and posterior surfaces. The posterior surface is nearly flat and can be easily palpated by rectal digital examination.

Hypertrophy of this gland is common in elder persons and may cause dysuria due to compression of the urethra.

4.6   Pelvic part of the ductus deferens

The ductus deferens is the duct carrying sperms from the testis to the ejaculatory duct.

4.7   Seminal vesicle

4.8   Ejaculatory duct

It is formed by the junction of the excretory duct of the seminal vesicle and the terminal portion of ampulla ductus deferentis at the neck of bladder. It is about 2 cm long, pass through the prostatic tissue and ends by entering the urethra on the seminal colliculus beside the prostatic utricle.

4.9   Uterus

4.9.1   Position, shape and relations

The uterus is pear-shaped. It has anterior, posterior surfaces and two lateral borders. It can be divided into fundus, body, isthmus and neck(cervix).

4.9.2   Ligaments

The ligaments of uterus including the broad ligament of uterus and the cardinal ligament of uterus.

4.9.3   Blood supply

● Uterine artery   It comes from the internal iliac artery and descends in front of the ureter to the base of the broad ligament of uterus.

● Uterine vein   It emerges from the uterovaginal venous plexus and joins the internal iliac vein.

4.9.4   Nerves

The sympathetic and parasympathetic nerves from the uterovaginal plexus are distributed to the body and neck of uterus.

4.10   Ovaries

They are oval-shaped which is about 3 cm in length, 1.5 cm in width and 1 cm thickness. It attached one on each side to the back of the broad ligament of uterus by the mesovarium. They have superior and inferior extremities, anterior and posterior borders and medial and lateral surfaces.

4.11   Uterine tubes

Each tube occupies the free edge of the broad ligament of uterus. It is about 8~12 cm in length, extending from the uterus upward and laterally to the inferior extremity of the ovary, then, along its anterior border, curves backward over the superior extremity to the medial surface of the ovary. Each orifice has four parts and two orifices: the uterine part, isthmus, ampulla and infundibulum, the abdominal orifice and the uterine orifice.

4. 12　Vagina

It is a muscular membranous tubes situated in the middle part of the pelvis. Its anterior and posterior walls are applied to each other. The lower part of the neck of uterus projects into a slightly enlarged upper part of the cavity of the vagina, and separates the vaginal walls.

Section 2 Dissection and observation

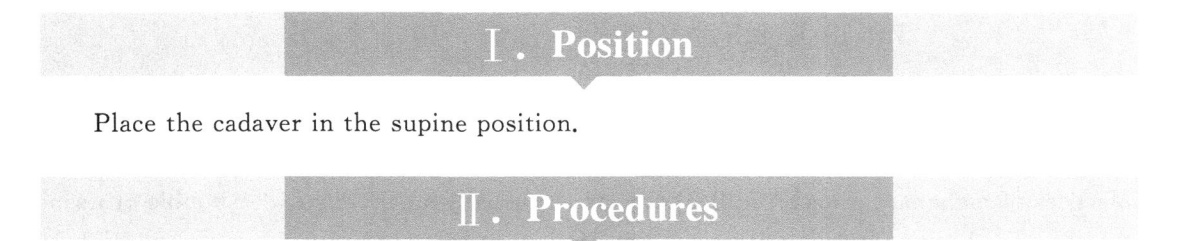

Ⅰ. Position

Place the cadaver in the supine position.

Ⅱ. Procedures

1 Dissect the major vessels in the pelvis

In the left iliac fossa, turn the sigmoid colon to the left. Along the right surface of the sigmoid mesocolon, cut through the peritoneum and remove it to find the inferior mesenteric artery. Clean its terminal branch—the superior rectal artery to the pelvis; remove its accompanying vein. Pull the rectum forward, clean the branches of the superior rectal artery to the side of rectum. Next, along the middle portion of the anterior surface of sacrum, find and clean the median sacral artery.

In the male pelvis, remove the peritoneum on the lateral wall of the pelvis, then at the deep inguinal ring, find the spermatic cord and separate the ductus deferens from the testicular vessels, trace these vessels to the upper margin of the greater pelvis.

In the female pelvis, find the ovary in the ovarian fossa or on the back of the broad ligament of uterus. Along the upper end of ovary, find the suspensory ligament of ovary. Cut through the peritoneum here, find the ovarian vessels and trace them to the ovary and uterine tube. Lateral to the neck of uterus, cut the peritoneum of broad ligament to find the ureter, separate it from the uterine artery which crosses it anterosuperiorly. Clean the uterine artery to its origin, and trace it along the lateral side of the uterus. Dissect the other blood vessels using the same procedures as in the dissection of male pelvis.

2 Dissect the sacral plexus

Trace the lumbosacral trunk downward along the medial side of the psoas major. Find the sacral plexus in front of the piriformis and deep to the internal iliac artery. Trace the components of the sacral plexus to the anterior sacral foramina.

Observe the pelvic sympathetic trunk and pelvic plexus.

Section 3

Clinical application

I. Ovarian cysts

Ovarian cysts generally occur either in the follicles or within the corpus luteum. Although most ovarian cysts are not dangerous, they must be examined thoroughly as possible sites of malignant cancer. Follicular cysts are usually small, distended bubble of tissue that are filled with fluid. Ordinarily, small follicular cysts are asymptomatic unless they rupture, but large or multiple cysts may cause pelvic pain, hematuria and irregular ovulation. In menopausal women, follicular cysts secret excessive estrogen in response for increased LH and FSH secretion.

II. Prostatic cancer

Prostatic cancer is one of the most common cancer in the males. Most prostatic cancers originate in the posterior portion of the gland. When the cancer spreads beyond the prostate, it usually travels along the ejaculatory ducts in the spaces between the seminal vesicles. Because prostatic cancer rarely onset of symptoms. Until they are well advanced, prostatic cancer is often fatal. Annual or semiannual digital rectal examination may detect small, hard nodule while it is still limited, and in such cases the recovery rate is high. Regular examinations are quite important for men over 40.

III. Pelvic inflammatory disease

Pelvic inflammatory disease (PID) is a general term referring inflammation of the uterus and uterine tubes with or without inflammation of the ovary, including localized pelvic peritonitis and abscess formation. It is the most severe complication of the sexually transmitted diseases caused by *N. Gonorrhoeae* and *C. trachomatis*. The infection can be controlled with antibiotics, if treatment is begun early. Severe cases of PID can lead to peritonitis.

Ⅳ. Fracture of the pelvis

Fracture of the pelvis is not common, although the pelvis may stand large forge, violence can still cause fracture of the pelvis. The weak areas of the pelvis are: the sacroiliac area, the ala of the ilium and the pubic rami. The fractures of pubic-obturator area are common and usually very complex. The direct violence may lead to fractures of sacrum, iliac crest or the other part of the pelvis which often combines with injuries to the pelvic organs, i. e. the rupture of urinary bladder and urethra may cause extravasation of urine; massive hemorrhage may happened if great blood vessels are injured by fracture.

Section 4

Ask yourself

1. What two arteries are divisions of the common iliac artery? Explain their branches and distributions.

2. Explain the position, shape, relation and the ligaments of the uterus.

3. Explain the relations of the rectum and the significance of rectal digital examination?

Chapter 8

The perineum

Section 1

Review

I. Surface anatomy

The perineum is the part of trunk below the pelvic diaphragm. It has the same boundaries as the outlet of pelvis extending from the lower border of the pubic symphysis to the coccyx. Its lateral boundaries are the inferior rami of the pelvis, the rami of ischia and sacrotuberous ligaments, a line joining the anterior parts of the ischial tuberosities divides the perineum into a large posterior anal region and a small anterior urogenital region.

II. Boundaries and divisions

The lateral boundaries of the perineum are the inferior rami of the pubes, the rami of ischia and the sacrotuberous ligaments. The perineum contains a large posterior anal region and a small anterior urogenital region by a line joining the anterior parts of the ischial tubersities.

III. Main contents

1 The anal region

The subcutaneous tissue of this region extends upward on both sides of anal canal to fill the ischiorectal fossa and allows distension of the anal canal.

1.1 Anal canal

This canal extends posteroinferiorly from the lower end of the pelvic part of the return to the anus. It is 3~4 cm long, and is surrounded by the sphincter ani internus and exernus.

● Sphincter ani internus   It is the thickened inner circular smooth muscle around the upper two thirds of the anal canal.

● Sphincter ani externus   It has three parts which are distinctly separated from each other. The subcutaneous part surrounds the anus. The superficial part is oval in shape, its fibers arise from the coccyx and pass anteriorly around the anus to the perineal central tendon. The deep part is fused with the puborectal part of the levator ani which reinforces its action.

1. 2   Ischioanal (ischiorectal) fossa

This wedge-shaped space situates lateral to the anus and rectum and is filled with fat. Its apex lies superiorly,and the base is the perineal skin. The lateral wall is formed by the ischial tuberosity, the sacrotuberous ligament and the fascia of obturator internus. Posteriorly of the fossa is bounded by the gluteus maximus and the sacrotuberous ligament. This fossa extends forward above the urogenital diaphragm and backward deep to the gluteus maximus. These two extensions are called the anterior and posterior recess respectively. The ischioanal fossa contains the branches of the pudendal nerve and internal pudendal vessels.

1. 3   Blood supply, nerves and lymphatic drainage

The pudendal nerve and the internal pudendal vessels leave the pelvis through the lesser sciatic foramen, and enter the pudendal canal. In the pudendal canal, the anal artery, vein and nerve are given off at once from the neuro-vascular bundle. They break into multiple branches to supply the perineal skin and the anal canal. In the anterior part of the anal region, the pudendal nerve and the internal pudendal artery divide into the dorsal nerve and arteries of penis(or clitoris) and the perineal nerve and artery.

2   Urogenital region in the male

This region is bounded anteriorly by the pubic symphysis, laterally by the ischiopubic rami and posteriorly by the line passing between the anterior part of the ischial tuberosities.

2. 1   Superficial structures

In this region, there are three layers of fascia separated by superficial and deep perineal spaces with their contents. The superficial fascia can be divided into two layers, the superficial layer is fatty layer, the deep layer is membranous layer called superficial fascia of perineum, or known as Colles' fascia. It is continuous anteriorly with the Scarpa's fascia of the abdominal wall, the dartos coat of the scrotum, and the superficial fascia of the penis. Laterally it is attached to the pubic arches and ischial tuberosities. The other two layers of fascia in this region are the inferior and superior fasciae of the urogenital diaphragm.

2. 2   Deep structures

● Superficial perineal space   It is the space between the Colles' fascia and the inferior fascia of urogenital diaphragm. It contains the superficial transverse muscle of perineum, the crura of penis, the ischiocavernosus, the bulbocaverous and the bulb of urethra (penis) as well as the perineal vessels and nerve.

● Deep perineal space   It is the portion enclosed between the inferior fascia of urogenital diaphragm and superior fascia of urogenital diaphragm. It contains the membranous part of urethra, the sphincter of urethra and the bulbourethral glands. The deep transverse muscle of perineum lies in it posteriorly.

● Urogenital diaphragm   It is formed basically by the sphincter of urethra, the deep transverse muscle of perineum, and the superior and inferior fascia of urogenital diaphragm.

● Perineal central tendon (perineal body)   This indefinite mass of fibrous tissue lies between the anal canal and the bulb of urethra. It gives attachments to the muscles of perineum.

2.3   The scrotum

A fibromuscular sac containing the testes, epididymises and lower parts of the spermatic cords, hangs below the pubic symphysis between the anteromedial aspects of the thighs. It is divided into right and left compartments by the septum of scrotum.

2.4   The spermatic cord

As the testis traverses the abdominal wall into the scrotum in fetus, it carries its vessels, nerves and ductus deferens with it. These meet at the deep inguinal ring to form the spermatic cord, suspending the testis in the scrotum and extending from the deep inguinal ring to the posterior aspect of the testis. The internal spermatic fascia is a thin, loose layer around the spermatic cord, derived from the transversalis fascia.

2.5   The penis

It is composed of three cylindrical masses of erectile tissue. The two dorsally located masses are called cavernous body of penis, its posterior part is called crus penis which is attached on the pubic arch. The single smaller ventral mass, the cavernous body of urethra contains the spongy part of the urethra. It is expanded at the distal end to form the glans penis, its posterior end becomes the bulb of urethra.

The superficial dorsal vein of penis lies in the superficial fascia in the median plane and drains into either the right or left external pudendal vein. The deep dorsal vein, also in the median plane but deep to the deep fascia of penis, passes between the lamellae of the suspensory ligament below the infrapubic ligament to drain into the pudendal and prostatic plexuses. Two dorsal arteries, the terminal branches of the internal pudendal artery, course lateral to the deep dorsal vein and supply the albuginea of cavernous body of penis, fascia of penis and the skin. The dorsal arteries are accompanied by two dorsal nerves, the terminal branches of the pudendal nerve, which course lateral to the dorsal arteries and supply twigs to the skin of the penis.

2.6   The male urethra

It is 16~20 cm in length which begins at the neck of urinary bladder and opens at the external orifice of urethra. The male urethra is subdivided into three parts-prostatic, membranous and cavernous.

The prostatic part of urethra is approximately 3 cm long. It begins at the neck of bladder and traverses the prostate. It ends at the superior fascia of the urogenital diaphragm.

The membranous part of urethra is the shortest (1 – 2 cm), the thinnest, the narrowest and the least dilatable part. It is within the urogenital diaphragm and surrounded by the sphincter of urethra.

The cavernous part of urethra is embedded in the cavernous body of urethra.

3　Urogenital region in the female

In the female, many structures in this region are similar to those in the male. It has the same layers as following, from superficial to deep, the skin, the superficial fascia of perineum, superficial perineal muscles, inferior fascia of urogenital diaphragm, deep perineal muscle, and superior fascia of urogenital diaphragm. The differences between the female and male in this region are as follows: in the female, the superficial perineal space contains, the crura of clitoris, the bulbs of vestibule and greater vestibular glands.

The female urethra is 3 – 5 cm long and very dilatable, extends from the neck of bladder passing through the pelvic cavity and the urogenital diaphragm, and opens immediately anterior to the vaginal orifice. Throughout its length, it is attached to the anterior wall of the vagina. Most of its lining is stratified squamous or columnar epithelium, and a number of small mucous glands open into it.

Section 2

Dissection and observation

I. Position and incisions

Place the body in the prone position. Make a median line position incision from the tip of coccyx, skirt around the anus, to the bottom of the scrotum. Then turn over the body and continue the incision around the scrotum or the greater lips of the pudendum to the pubic symphysis.

II. Procedures

Remove or turn over the skin laterally to the thigh and the gluteal region.

1 Dissect the anal region

Remove the fatty tissue from the ischiorectal fossa by forceps, find the pudendal canal on the lateral wall. Cut the medial wall of this canal. Identify and clean the pudendal vessels and their branches.

Remove the fascia from the sphincter ani externus which surrounds the anus.

Take away the remaining fat from the ischiorectal fossa, expose this wedge-shaped space. Observe the subcutaneous, the superficial and deep parts of the sphincter ani externus. Find that the anterior recess of the ischiorectal fossa and the posterior recess of the ischiorectal fossa.

2 Dissect the urogenital region

Make a median longitudinal incision the skin of the rahpe of scrotum, turn over the skin laterally. Cut the dartos on the median line and cut the superficial fascia of perineum (Colles' fascia) from the posterior end of the median scrotal incision to the ischial tuberosity.

Remove the Colles' fascia to expose the structures in the superficial perineal space. Find the cutaneous branches of the perineal nerve which arises from the pudendal nerve, and find the branches of the perineal artery from the internal pudendal artery.

2.1 Examine the muscles in the superficial perineal space

The bulbocavemosus in the male pass anterosuperiorly round each side of the bulb of urethra from the raphe penis. They insert into the upper surface of the bulb of urethra and the cavernous body of penis. In the female, the muscles are smaller and surround the side of the vaginal vestibule from the perineal central tendon to the crura of clitoris. The ischiocavernosus covers the inferior surface of each crus of cavernous body of penis of clitoris.

2.2 Remove the superficial perineal muscles

Expose the bulb of urethra or the bulbs of vestibule, the cavernous body of penis,and the crura of penis. The bulbs of vestibule lie on each side of the vaginal orifice. The greater vestibular glands are two in number and lie under the cover of posterior pole of the bulbs of vestibule. Each one has a long duct which opens at the side of the vaginal orifice between the hymen and the lesser lip of pudendum.

Detach crura of penis or clitoris from the ischiopubic rami, and the bulb of urethra(or bulbs of vestibule)from the deep fascia on the inferior surface of the urogenital diaphragm. Expose the deep fascia on the inferior surface of the urogenital diaphragm.

Remove the inferior fascia of urogenital diaphragm or reflect it anteriorly. Examine the contents in the deep perineal space. The artery and nerve to the penis or clitoris lie between them. In the male, find the artery to the penis, which is derived from the internal pudendal artery. Expose and trace the urethral bulbar artery. Try to find the bulbourethral glands, the ducts of them pierce the inferior fascia of urogenital diaphragm to open into the cavernous or spongy part of urethra.

Section 3

Clinical application

The uterine prolapse is an abnormal descending of the uterus, its cervix may descend below the level of ischial spine. In some marked cases, the cervix may protrude through the vaginal orifice. The uterine prolapse occurs most commonly as a result of childbirth which injures the fixative and supporting structures, such as the ligaments, pelvic diaphragm, urogenital diaphragm and perineal body. The other etiology which may lead to prolapse are relaxation of connective tissues in elder persons or a retroversion position of the uterus.

Section 4

Ask yourself

1. Depict the spermatic cord and its coverings.
2. If the rupture of the urethra occurs, explain the reason of the urinary extravasation.
3. What are the superficial perineal space and the deep perineal space?
4. How does the male urethra divide?
5. Describe the ischioanal fossa and its clinical significance.

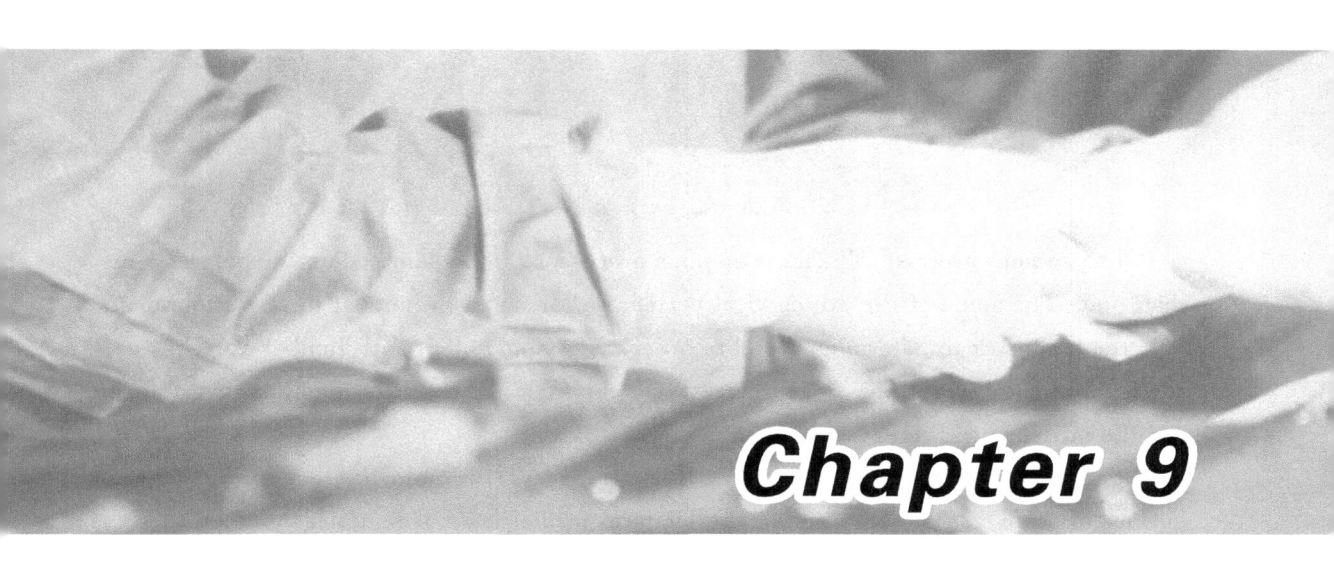

Chapter 9

The back and the vertebral region

Section 1

Review

Ⅰ. Surface anatomy

The **spinous process**   The most spinous processes can be palpated on the posterior median line. The spine of the 7th cervical vertebra is the most prominent in all vertebrae and it is the landmark to determine vertebra order. The spine of the 4th lumbar vertebra is at the level of the highest point of iliac crest and the sacral spines fuse together finally forming the median sacral crest.

The **spine of scapula and acromion**   It is a transverse, prominent crest on the posterior surface of scapula. The line linking the bilateral medial ends of scapular spine crosses the 3rd thoracic spine. The lateral end is called acromion and its tip is the highest point on the shoulder.

The **inferior angle of scapula**   It is opposite to the 7th rib or 7th intercostal space when the upper limb is downward.

The **twelfth rib**   It can be palpated in the lateral side of erector spinae at the lower border of thorax.

The **erector spinae and vertebrocostal angle**   It can be palpated in the lateral sides of spine. Renal angle is located between lateral border of erector spinae and the 12th rib.

The **iliac crest and posterior superior iliac spine**   The iliac crest, with an "S" shape in whole length, is the upper border of iliac ala. The posterior superior iliac spine is a sharp projection of posterior end of iliac crest whereas it appears a fossa on the surface of skin.

The **sacral hiatus and sacral cornu**   Along the median sacral crest downward, there is a foramen that is the inferior orifice of the vertebral canal is named sacral hiatus. The sacral cornu is a pair of prolonged tubercle on both sides of sacral hiatus which is easily palpated on surface, through which local anesthetic may be injected into the sacral canal.

The **coccyx**   It can be palpated inferior to the apex of sacrum.

II . Boundaries and divisions

The superior boundary of the back and vertebral region is the external occipital protuberance and the superior nuchal line. Its inferior boundary is the line from the apex of coccyx to the posterior superior iliac spine. Its lateral boundary is the anterior border of trapezius, the posterior border of deltoid, and the posterior axillary line. It could be divided into the nape, the back, the lumbar and the sacrococcygeal regions.

III . Main contents

1　Skin

It is thicker and abundant of tight connection with superficial fascia, so it is difficult to separate, especially in the nape.

2　Superficial fascia

It is thicker and tighter, particular in the upper portion of nape. There are many fibrous fibers connecting to the deep superficial fascia, and superficial blood vessels, cutaneous nerves as well as superficial lymph vessels in it. The superficial fascia contains two layers, and there are lot of areolar connective tissues between them in lumbar region.

All cutaneous nerves are the branches of the dorsal rami of the spinal nerves which pierce the muscles 2 cm lateral to the posterior median line. The main cutaneous nerves in nape are the greater occipital nerve and the 3rd occipital nerve. The superior clunial nerves are the branches of dorsal rami of the upper three lumbar nerves. They pierce the deep fascia over the iliac crest at the lateral margin of erector spinae, and slope downward to the gluteal region.

The superficial blood vessels in the back and lumbar region are thin. The arteries are the branches of the posterior intercostal arteries and the posterior branches of lumbar arteries. Those blood vessels are accompanied by corresponding cutaneous nerves.

3　Deep fascia

It envelopes the surface of muscles and separates the muscles of different layers. The deep fascia of nape is a part of the superficial lamina of the deep cervical fascia and encloses the trapezius.

In the lumbar region, the thoracolumbar fascia is divided into three layers.

The posterior layer is the thickest layer which situated posteriorly to the erector.

The middle layer is located between the erector spinae and the quadrates lumborum. It

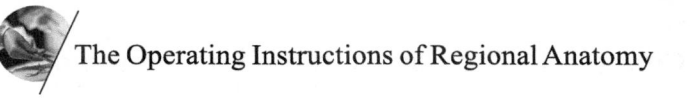

unites with the posterior layer at the lateral margin of the erector spinae, finally forms the sheath of the erector spinae with the posterior layer together. At the lateral border of the quadrates lumborum, it also forms the aponeurotic origin of the transversus abdominis.

The anterior layer covers the quadratus lumborum anteriorly and is also named the fascia of quadratus lumborum.

4 Muscles

The muscles of the back can be divided into four layers. The first layer includes the trapezius, the latissimus dorsi and the posterior part of the obliquus externus abdominis. The second layer contains the splenius capitis, the semispinalis capitis, the levator scapulae and the rhomboideus in nape, the serratus posterior superior, the serratus posterior inferior and the posterior part of the obliquus internus abdominis in back of the thorax. The third layer muscles are the erector spinae and the posterior part of the transversus abdominis. The fourth layer includes a group of suboccipital muscles (located between the first, the second cervical vertebra and the occipital) in nape, the quadratus lumborum and the psoas major in lumbar as well as some short muscles lateral to the spine.

5 Triangles of the back and nape

● Superior lumbar triangle   It is bounded by the serratus posterior inferior, the erector spinae and the obliquus internus abdominis. In the depth of this triangle, it is passed by the subcostal, the iliohypogastric and the ilioinguinal nerves.

● Inferior lumbar triangle   It is limited by the lower part of the lateral margin of the lasttissimus dorsi, the posterior free border of the obliquus externus abdominis and the iliac crest.

● Suboccipital triangle   It is bounded medially by the rectus capitis posterior major, laterally by the obliquus capitis superior, and inferiorly by the obliquus capitis inferior. It contains the vertebral artery and suboccipital nerve and vessels.

● Triangle of auscultation   It is formed by the latissimus dorsi, trapezius and the medial border of the scapula. This triangle is free of overlying muscles and suited to auscultate the breathing sounds.

In the posterior median line, the layers from surface to deep are skin, superficial fascia, supraspinal ligament, interspinal ligament, ligament flava, lamina of vertebral arch, vertebral canal.

Table 8 – 1 The comparation of layers of the medial and the lateral lumbar region

Medial	Lateral
Skin	Skin
Superficial fascia	Superficial fascia
Deep fascia	Deep fascia
The aponeurosis of latissimus dorsi The posterior layer of thoracolumbar fascia	The latissimus dorsi The obliquus externus abdominis The inferior lumbar triangle
The erector spinae The middle layer of thoracolumbar fascia	The obliquus internus abdominis The serratus posterior inferior The superior lumbar triangle The transversus abdominis and its fascia, with the subcostal nerve, the iliohypogastric nerve and the ilioinguinal nerve deep to it
The psoas major and its fascia The quadratus lumborum and its fascia	The transverse fascia

1.6 Vertebral canal and its contents

1.6.1 Vertebral canal

It is formed by the vertebral foramina of 24 movable vertebral bones, sacral canal of the sacral bone and the joints between the vertebrae. It contains the spinal cord, the roots of spinal nerves and spinal meninges and vessels.

Superiorly—continued with cranial cavity by the foramen magnum.

Inferiorly—opening at the back of sacral bone by sacral hiatus.

Anteriorly—formed by the posterior aspect of vertebral bodies, intervertebral discs and the posterior longitudinal ligament.

Posteriorly—formed by the laminae of vertebral arches and ligamenta flava.

Laterally—formed by the pedicles of the vertebral arches and the intervertebral foramina.

1.6.2 Spinal meninges and space

● Dura mater It is a tough, fibrous, outermost layer of the meninges. It continues with the dura mater of the brain at the foramen magnum superiorly; laterally continues with the external membrane of the spinal nerve; and inferiorly encloses the terminal filum and is attached to the back of coccyx.

● Arachnoid mater It is a filmy, transparent, spidery layer connected to the pia mater by web-like trabeculations.

● Pia mater   It is a delicate, vascular membrane which closely attached to the surface of spinal cord and dives into the fissures and sulci of the spinal cord.

● Epidural space   It is external to the dura mater and contains the internal vertebral venous plexus, lymphatic vessels and epidural fat. Clinically, local anaesthetic can be injected into this space to block the conduction of the spinal nerves.

● Subarachnoid space   It is between the arachnoid and the pia mater and filled with cerebrospinal fluid (CSF). The enlarged subarachnoid space between vertebrae L1 and S2 is named the terminal cistern.

Section 2

Dissection and observation

Place the cadaver in the prone position and put a steel pillow under the sternoclavicular joint in order to slightly bend the neck anteriorly.

Palpate the markers such as the external occipital protuberance, the mastoid process, the spinous processes of the 7th cervical vertebra, the thoracic and lumbar vertebrae, the acromion, the spine of scapula, the iliac crest and so on.

Make the following incisions:

● A median vertical incision from the external occipital protuberance to the spinous process of the 5th lumbar vertebra.

● The superior transverse incision from the external occipital protuberance to the base of the mastoid process.

● The inferior transverse incision from the spinous process of the 7th cervical verterbra to the acromion.

● A curve incision, from the spinous process of the 5th lumbar vertebra along the iliac crest to the anterior superior iliac spine, should be made if the skin of the gluteal region is not incised.

II. Procedures

1 Dissect the superficial structures

Beginning in the median line, turn all the skin flaps laterally.

Find the cutaneous nerves near the paravertebral line (about 2~3 cm laterally to the median line) as they pierce the deep fascia. They are the branches of the dorsal rami of the spinal nerves. The superior 6 pairs of branch of the thoracic nerves go to the lateral horizontally. However, in the lower thoracic and lumbar regions, these branches descend before they reaching the skin.

Find the greater occipital nerve as it appears 2~3 cm lateral to the external occipital protuberance with the occipital artery laterally. The 3rd occipital nerve is located in the superficial fascia and between the median plane and the greater occipital nerve.

Try to find the cutaneous branches of the dorsal rami of the upper three lumbar nerves. They pierce the deep fascia a short distance superior to the iliac crest and go down over it to supply the skin of the gluteal region.

2 Dissect the deep structures

2.1 Dissect the deep fascia on the surface of muscles

Clean the superficial and deep fascia from the surface of trapezius, latissimus dorsi. Pay attention to the accessory nerve at the lateral border of trapezius in the nape. Please reserve the thoracolumbar fascia, one part of the origin of the latissimus dorsi, during clean of the deep fascia. Find and expose the posterior border of obliquus externus abdominis at the lateral of the lumbar region.

2.2 Dissect the first layer of the muscles and the triangles bounded by them

This layer of muscles contains trapezius, latissimus dorsi and obliquus externus abdominis. Observe and review the formation, origin, insertion and function of trapezius, latissimus dorsi. Identify the triangle of auscultation bounded by the lateral lower border of trapezius, the superior border of latissimus dorsi, and the spinal border of the scapula. Another is the inferior lumbar triangle bounded by the lower part of the lateral margin of the lastissimus dorsi, the iliac crest and the posterior border of obliquus externus abdominis.

Insert the handle of scalpel into the deep of trapezius at the lateral lower margin and separate the muscle medially to its origin (the spinous processes of the thoracic vertebrae). Then cut trapezius 2 cm lateral to the posterior median line and reflect the muscle laterally, do not damage the occipital artery, greater occipital nerve, spinal accessory nerve, levator scapulae and rhomboidei.

Clean the inferior border of latissimus dorsi and bluntly separate it medially and inferiorly to the thoracolumbar fascia. Transect the muscle 1 cm lateral to the junction of the belly and the aponeurosis, and reflect the flaps laterally. Look for the serratus posterior inferior that is on the deep of latissimus dorsi.

2.3 Dissect the second layer of muscles and the superior lumbar triangle

The second layer of muscles includes splenius, semispinalis capitis, levator scapulae, rhomboidei, serratus posterior inferior, serratus posterior superior and the posterior part of the obliquus internus abdominis. Find the dorsal scapular nerve which supplies levator scapulae and rhomboidei, and the accompanying vessels at the anterior margin of levator scapulae.

2.3.1   Dissect the rhomboidei

Identify its origins from the spinous processes of the 6th, 7th cervical and the upper four thoracic vertebrae. Cut through the rhomboidei near its origins and turn this muscle laterally. Then, observe the serratus posterior superior, look for the dorsal scapular artery and nerve.

2.3.2   Dissect the serratus posterior superior

Cut the serratus posterior superior 1 cm lateral to the posterior median line and turn it laterally. Now observe the origin and insertion of the splenius capitis and splenius cervicis, detach the two splenius muscles from the spinous processes of the vertebrae, and turn them laterally as far as you can, to reveal the semispinalis capitis. Clean the serratus posterior inferior at the junction of the back of thoracic region and the lumbar region. Then observe the insertion of the serratus posterior inferior on ribs and compare the direction of the serratus posterior inferior and the serratus posterior superior.

2.3.3   Dissect the superior lumbar triangle

It is usually bounded by the serratus posterior inferior, the erector spinae and the obliquus internus abdominis. The latissimus dorsi overlays this triangle and the transversus abdominis is its floor. This triangle will change into quadrangle if the inferior border of the 12th rib also bound this region. Identify the subcostal, iliohypogastric, and ilioinguinal nerves crossing the triangle.

2.3.4   Dissect the serratus posterior inferior

Cut the serratus posterior inferior at the origin and reflex laterally. Clean the aponeurosis of transversus abdominis and identify the tough lumbocostal ligament which is formed by the aponeurosis of transversus abdominis and located between the 12th rib and transverse process of the 1st lumbar vertebra.

Cut the aponeurosis of transversus abdominis at its lateral part and reflex medially. Expose the subcostal, iliohypogastric, and ilioinguinal nerves deeply to the aponeurosis. Finally, cut the posterior layer of renal fascia, the adipose capsule in order to reveal the kidney.

2.4   Dissect thoracolumbar fascia and the third layer muscles

2.4.1   Dissect and observe thoracolumbar fascia

The thoracolumbar fascia contains three layers and enclose the erector spinae and quadratus lumborum. Make a vertical incision through the middle of the posterior layer of the fascia from the 12th rib to the iliac crest. Turn the fascial flap laterally, and look for the erector spinae. Push the erector medially and explore the middle layer of the fascia by your fingers upward, downward and medially to its attachments.

2.4.2 Observe and review the erector spinae

The erector spinae is the largest group of intrinsic back muscles. The muscles lie posterolaterally to the vertebral column between the spinous processes medially and the angles of the ribs laterally. The mass arises from a broad, thick tendon attached to the sacrum, the spinous processes of the lumbar and lower thoracic vertebrae, and the iliac crest. It includes, in the upper lumbar region, three vertical columns of muscle, each of which is further subdivided regionally (lumborum, thoracis, cervicis and capitis), depending on the insertion. The outer or most laterally placed column of the erector spinae is the iliocostalis, which is associated with the costal elements and passes from the common tendon of origin to multiple insertions into the angles of the ribs and the transverse processes of the lower cervical vertebrae. The middle or intermediate column is the longissimus, which is the largest of the erector spinae subdivision extending from the common tendon of origin to the base of the skull. The most medial muscle is the spinalis, which is most constant in the thoracic region and is generally absent in the cervical region. It is united with a deeper muscle (the semispinalis capitis).

2.5 Dissect the fourth muscles and the suboccipital triangle

2.5.1 Dissect the fourth layer muscles

This group of muscles includes transversospinalis, intertransversarii, suboccipital muscles and so on. Remove the fibers of the erector spinae with tweezers, especially the spinalis and longissimus. Then dissect the three layers of fibers of the transversospinalis. The superficial fibers are semispinalis capitis and semispinalis cervicis, semispinalis thoracis. Remove the semispinalis thoracis to expose the multifidus muscle that belongs to the middle fibers. Finally remove the multifidus muscle to expose the deep fibers (rotator). The intertransversarii which between the adjacent transverse processes are remarkable in lumbar region. It is needed to only expose 1~2 intertransversarii in lumbar region.

2.5.2 Dissect and observe the suboccipital triangle

Observe the splenius capitis, the splenius cervicis and the levator scapulae. Cut the superior portion of this muscle and reflect it inferiorly, avoiding damage of the strong, posterior branch of the 2nd cervical spinal nerve (greater occipital nerve). Observe the suboccipital triangle which is bounded by two obliquus capitis and the rectus capitis posterior major. Next, look for the vertebral artery in the triangle. Inferiorly, the suboccipital nerve may be found which supplies the suboccipital muscles.

2.6 Dissect the vertebral canal

Remove the muscles of the back to expose the spinous processes and vertebral laminae of the lumbar and thoracic vertebrae. Divide the laminae of the vertebral arches close to the medial side of the articular process with a vertebral saw bilaterally. Remove the posterior wall of the vertebral canal and observe the strong and elastic yellow ligaments.

2.6.1　Identify the meninges of the spinal cord, the epidural space and the subarachnoid space.

Remove the fatty tissue and venous plexus in the vertebral canal to expose the dura mater of the spinal cord. Then, carefully cut the dura mater in the dorsal median line and protect the underlying arachnoid as possible as you can. Reflex the dura mater to reveal the arachnoid. Incise the arachnoid along the median line, and expose the spinal cord and its covering of pia mater. The spinal pia mater is thicker than that of the brain, and firmly adheres to the spinal cord. On each side of the spinal cord, look for the tooth-like projections of pia mater (the denticulate ligaments). The denticulate ligaments insert to the spinal dura mater are between the anterior and posterior rootlets of spinal nerves.

2.6.2　Observe the other contents in the vertebral canal

In the specimens, observe and review the follows: ① the spinal cord, especially its cervical and lumbar enlargements; ② the relationship of the level of the spinal cord and the vertebral body; ③ the filum terminale and its attachment; the terminal cistern of the spinal subarachnoid space and the cauda equina; ④ the spinal nerves, ventral and dorsal roots, ventral and dorsal rami of the spinal nerves, intervertebral disc and the posterior longitudinal ligament.

Section 3

Clinical application

Ⅰ. Herniated lumbar intervertebral disc

Due to the degeneration of the disc and the incorrect movement of the lumbar vertebrae, a rupture or protrusion of the lumbar intervertebral disc occurs and the nucleus pulposus herniates partially or completely into the spinal canal. Consequently, the roots of spinal nerves are impinged and irritated by the herniated disc resulting in a back pain or sciatica down to the lateral side of leg and into the sole of the foot.

The patients with herniated lumbar intervertebral disc are usually forced to bend their vertebral column laterally in order to relief the compression or irritation of the spinal nerve.

Ⅱ. Epidural anesthesia

It is widely used in surgery. The anesthetic agents are introduced into the epidural space where it diffuses through the connective tissue of the space, those block the nerves roots effectively. When using subarachnoid anesthesia, agents are introduced into the subarachnoid space where those mix with the cerebrospinal fluid and bath the spinal cord and nerve roots.

Ⅲ. Operative route for kidney in the loin

An oblique incision between the 12th rib and the iliac crest is usually used for the kidney operation. Latissimus dorsi and oliquus externus abdominis are cut and then serratus posterior inferior, then the 12th rib are exposed. Next obliquus internus abdominis and transversus abdominis are divided to reveal peritoneum anteriorly. The peritoneum is usually pushed forward. The renal fascial capsule is then clearly shown. If the 12th rib is needed to remove, more care must be taken to protect the pleura because it crosses the medial half of the 12th rib. At the same time it is necessary to protect the subcostal, iliohypogastric and ilioinguinal nerves.

Ⅳ. Lumbar spinal puncture

The extraction or sampling of CSF from the terminal cistern, is an important diagnostic method for evaluating a variety of central nervous system (CNS) disorders. Meningitis and diseases of the CNS may alter the cells in the CSF or change the concentration of its chemical constituents. Lumbar spinal puncture is performed with the patient leaning forward or lying on the side with the back flexed. Flexion of the vertebral column facilitates insertion of the needle by spreading the vertebral laminae and spinous processes apart, stretching the ligamenta flava.

Section 4

Ask yourself

1. Describe the distribution feature of the vessels and nerves on the back. Describe the origin and distribution of the main posterior branches of spinal nerves such as the greater occipital nerve and the superior clunial nerve.

2. Describe the distribution of the muscles on back, the structure and characteristic of the thoracolumbar fascia.

3. Describe the locations, boundaries and clinical significances of the suboccipital triangle, the auscultatory triangle, the superior lumbar triangle and the inferior lumbar triangle?

4. How to determine the position of puncture before the epidural anaesthesia, the subarachnoid anaesthesia or the extraction of the CSF is performed in the lumbar region? What are the layers of structure which are passed by the puncture needle?

5. Describe the surgical approach for kidney. And what layers of structure will be dealt with through this approach?

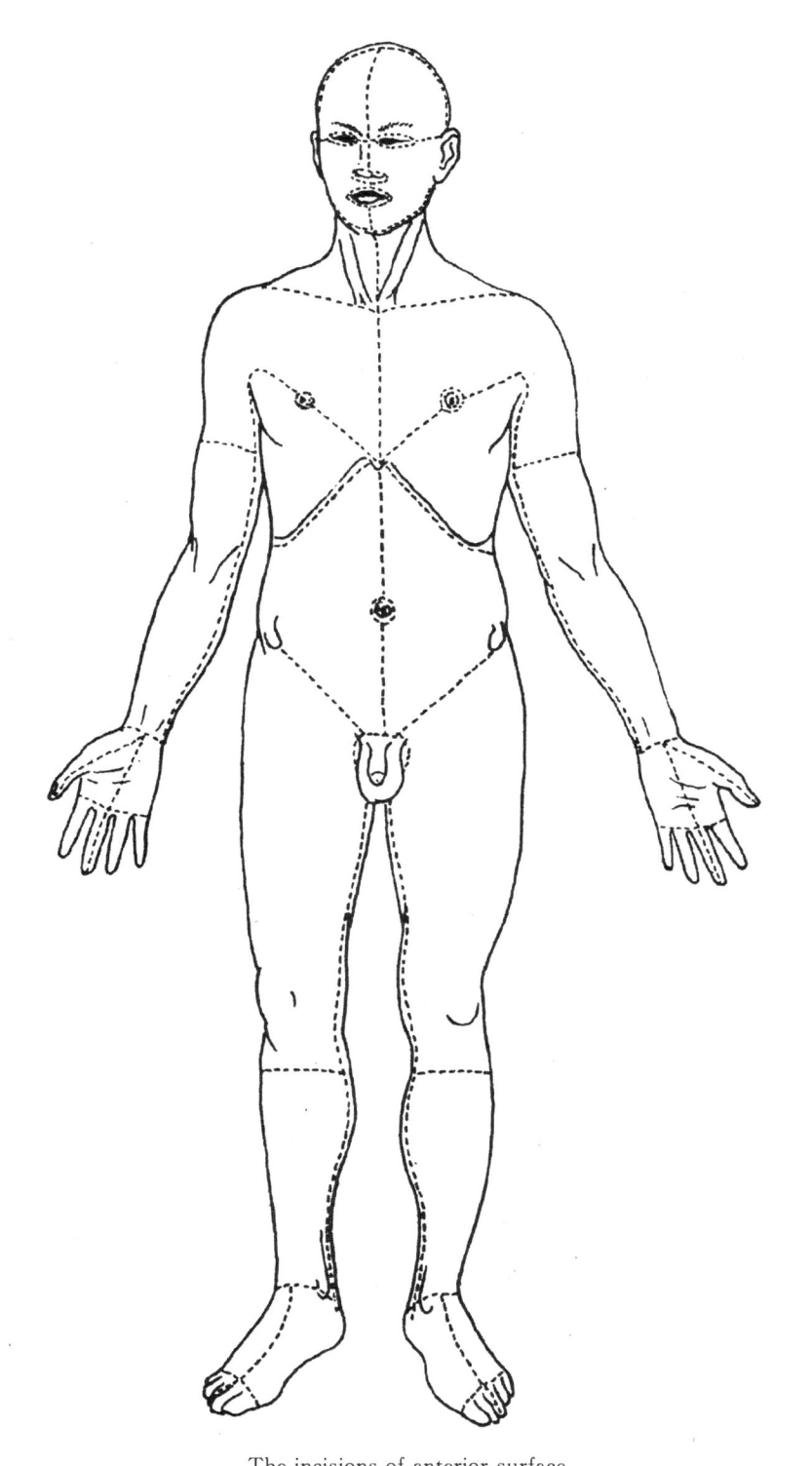

The incisions of anterior surface

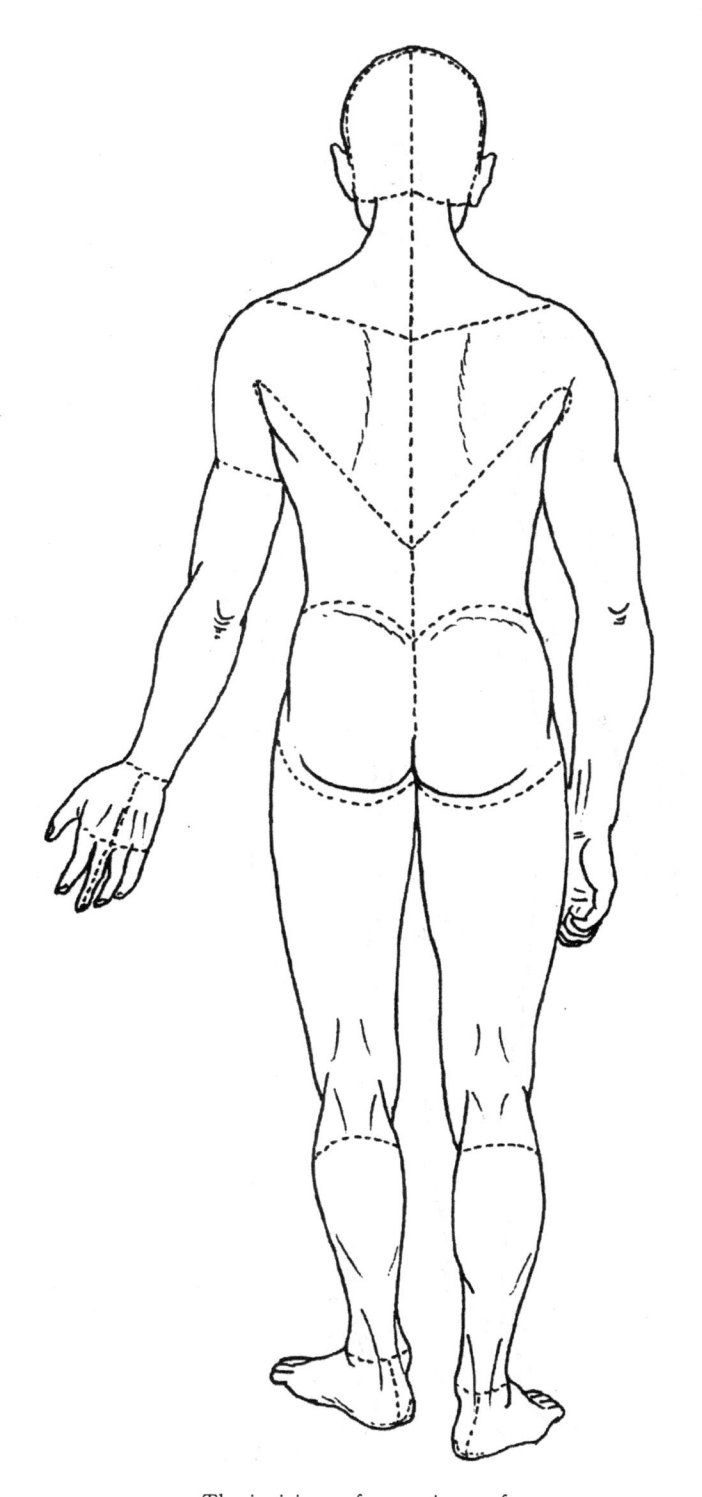

The incisions of posterior surface

Reference

1. Wang Huaijing, Liu Yong. Regional Anatomy. Changchun: Jilin Science and Technology Publishing Press, 2009.

2. Bo Shuling. Regional Anatomy. Beijing: People's Medical Publishing House Co, LTD, 2013.

3. Ronan O'Rahilly, Fabiola Muller, Stanley Carpenter, et al. Basic human anatomy: A regional study of human structure. Philadelphia: W. B. Saunders company, 1983.

4. Robert Carola, John P. Harley, Clarks R. Noback. Human Anatomy And Physiology. New York: McGraw—Hill, Inc, 1990.

5. Keith L. Moore, Arthur F. Dalley, Anne M. R. Agur. Clinically Oriented Anatomy. 6th Edition. Philadelphia: Lippincott Williams and Wilkins, 2009.

.